POLYMYALGIA RHEUMATICA AND GIANT CELL ARTERITIS – A SURVIVAL GUIDE

Dr. Kate Gilbert PhD.

ISBN: 1500713406
ISBN-13:9781500713409

DEDICATION

To my mother

CONTENTS

ACKNOWLEDGMENTS

This book would not have been possible without the help and active collaboration of so many of the remarkable clinicians and survivors of PMR and GCA I have met and worked with in recent years.

I have found the vast majority of clinical experts in the fields of rheumatology, ophthalmology and general practice, to be genuinely eager to share both their knowledge and the gaps in their knowledge with a demanding and opinionated layperson who will insist on asking awkward questions. Among them of course the outstanding example is Professor Bhaskar Dasgupta, who has devoted much of his career in rheumatology to solving the riddles of polymyalgia rheumatica and giant cell arteritis. His energy and enthusiasm are awe-inspiring, and thousands of PMR and GCA patients owe him a debt of gratitude for his dogged determination in bringing these profoundly unfashionable conditions to clinical and public notice.

Among other medical experts I must also mention with thanks Drs Colin Pease, Sarah Mackie, Kevin Barraclough, Brian Bourne, Toby Helliwell, Jane Gibson, Louise Warburton, Frances Borg; and Professors John Kirwan, Rashid Luqmani, Christian Mallen, Eoin O'Sullivan, Eric Matteson and Dennis McGonagle. Other researchers include Dr Sara Muller, Dr Helen Twohig, and Maggie Walsh.

Above all I thank my colleagues and friends in PMRGCAuk,

the trustees, support group organisers and volunteers who have all contributed to this work. Wendy Morrison, Jennifer Nott, Mavis Smith, Pam Hildreth, Margaret Wright, Lynne Boyle, Dorothy Byrne, Lady Wendy Levene, Laurene Brooks, Rob Murton, Robin Hamilton, Sarah Gray, Alison Jeffrey, Jean Miller, Bea Nicholson, Gillian Green, Christine Young, Catie Pickersgill, Clare Marshall, Shirley O'Connell, Ann Chambers, Dale Hodgson, Penny Denby, Hannah Padbury, Sue Halliday, Lorna Neill, Eric Clark, John Robson, Alan Walkington, Eileen Harrison: you are all part of the story and thank you so much for everything you have done, for the many thousands of PMR and GCA sufferers. Anything valuable in this book is thanks to you. Any errors, and of course all the opinions, are my own!

Finally my deepest appreciation for the many men and women who have shared with me their experiences of polymyalgia rheumatica and giant cell arteritis. Thanks to you, the struggle may not be so hard for those who come after you.

1. INTRODUCTION

One November morning, at the age of 54, I woke up with a searing pain in my shoulders and a strange feeling of paralysis. I stared at the ceiling for a while feeling terrified, and then set about hauling myself out of bed. I crashed into the bedroom wall and sat on the edge of the bed. "You've got *polymyalgia rheumatica*, like Mom had", I said to myself, as my memory dug up images of my mother struggling around the house 20 years before.

First off, having a long-term illness was not in my script. I thought I was doing all the right things; keeping fit, active, keeping the weight under control. One thing I had not been keeping under control as I got into my 50s was stress. Looking back, I can see that stress had been piling up on me from all directions. We had moved to Italy to start a new life. Then in 2004, we took the plunge and set up our permanent home there. We sold our beloved Victorian family house, where the children had grown up. We bought a new unfurnished apartment near Milan, and set about making it our new nest. It was just a concrete shell, and all the work of arranging the finishing, installing the plumbing, talking to builders, choosing floors and so on, fell to me, who had not had a word of Italian before we started. It was all a wonderful adventure and we were like a pair of newly-weds.

I would not change a minute of that experience, but I was not paying attention to the toll it was taking on my health. The month we moved in, my husband's company suggested that they wanted to 'change direction' and that his position was no longer secure. Things were not going to be as expected. As a middle-aged British woman, I was not going to break into the closed world that is the Italian university system. I went back to the UK to work, as a head of department in a Midlands university. I wasn't a popular choice for the job, and I knew it – the department had a favoured internal candidate and they weren't at all happy to have to work with me instead.

There followed two years of struggle and isolation, during which I was making the most of Ryanair's cheap fares by going 'home' to Milan every couple of weeks to see my man, who was trying to set himself up with a new career. Somewhere in the middle of it all, our daughter gave birth to our first grandchild by Caesarean section after four gruelling days of labour. Looking back, it is not surprising I got ill.

Now completely recovered (I haven't taken any medication for PMR for four years), I can look back and see how this experience of having a chronic inflammatory illness changed my life, in some ways for the worst, in other ways for the better. This book is a commitment to share with you what I have learned from this experience, but above all from the hundreds of people I have met with PMR or GCA.

The chances are that you are reading this book because you have been diagnosed either with Polymyalgia Rheumatica (PMR) or Giant Cell Arteritis (GCA, sometimes known as temporal arteritis, or TA). If you are particularly unlucky, with both. Chances are, too, that you had not heard of either of these before finding out that you have one of them. In a way, I was fortunate in having some prior experience. With this book, my aim is to inform you about PMR and GCA, realistically, and help you to know what to expect, without either being falsely optimistic or unduly pessimistic. The first thing you need to know about PMR and GCA is that you have an excellent chance of getting better. You may be feeling lousy at the moment because you are in the early stages. You may be a year or so into your condition and wondering whether it is ever going to end.

This idea of a duel with a dragon came to me one day when I started thinking about this book. Living with PMR or GCA, or if you have the double whammy, both of them, is a bit like fighting a dragon. Imagine a dragon with terrifying, staring eyes, breathing fire and smoke, consuming everything that stands in its way. That fiery head is like the acute phase when we first fall ill with PMR or GCA. See how the dragon has a long, sloping, spiny back, going up and down with spikes. That is like the long period when we are trying to recover, 'tapering' the steroids, and perhaps having difficulty, with one flare-up after another. The dosage of medication goes up and down, our symptoms go up and down, and finding the right balance between the two is a long and tedious struggle. Then see the dragon's tail. That has a sharp point that can take you by surprise. Just when you thought you had that dragon beat, up comes the tail to sting you with that barb. That is the sting in the tail of PMR or GCA. The years on steroids can leave you with an unwelcome reminder, in the form of injuries to your tendons and ligaments, or perhaps Type 2 diabetes. More about that later.

Polymyalgia Rheumatica and Giant Cell Arteritis are regarded as separate illnesses. However, they are categorized together because there is a significant overlap between them. It is estimated (Smeeth *et al,* 2006) that there are about 40,000 new cases of PMR and 10,000 new cases of GCA a year in the UK. Around one in five people with PMR also has GCA, while approximately four out of ten people with GCA also have the symptoms of PMR. For many years, the underlying reason for this overlap has been a bit of a medical mystery.

In recent years, more and more evidence is emerging that PMR, particularly the more complex cases, and GCA are both linked to, or different manifestations of, large vessel vasculitis, or inflammation in the large blood vessels of the body. In GCA, it is arteries in the neck and head that are most affected. In PMR, it is arteries feeding blood to the large muscles in the body. This is a simplified statement of a really complex situation.

There is still a whole lot that is unknown about PMR and

GCA. They have not been the subject of a great deal of research interest in the past. We need to have a look at the reasons for this relative neglect in order to understand how these diseases are diagnosed and treated. Nevertheless, we can say with confidence that there is a renewed interest in PMR and GCA in clinical research, and we can look forward to some major breakthroughs in knowledge in the near future.

We get going in Chapter 2 by taking a look at polymyalgia rheumatica (PMR), in some respects a less dangerous condition than GCA, but one that is largely misunderstood and underestimated by many doctors. Underestimated because they have little experience of what it is actually like living with this condition, and crucially, with the treatment. PMR attacks elderly people. The average age of onset is around 72 years. PMR also affects mainly women. Let us face it, elderly women are not the highest priority when it comes to medical care and cutting-edge research.

Chapter 3 focuses on Giant Cell Arteritis, what it is, and why it is so important to diagnose and treat quickly. GCA is the less common of the two conditions, and yet much more risky, seeing as the worst case scenario of the patient losing the sight of both eyes is catastrophic, irreversible, and potentially completely preventable. If you have been diagnosed with GCA, this chapter should give you information and also some reassurance that, once you are in treatment, the chance of this happening to you is infinitesimally small. I recommend that, even if you only have PMR on its own, or GCA on its own, that you read both chapter 1 and chapter 2, as there is information in each that everybody needs to know.

We move on in Chapter 4 to the thorny issue of treatment. This can be a very hard time for many sufferers, not least because the steroid treatment has the effect of filling out all our wrinkles and giving a lovely bloom to our skin. It is confusing and, frankly, wearing, to have friends and family exclaim 'Oh you do look well!' when you are feeling like crawling under a stone and not coming out again. The chapter deals with the challenges of tapering down dosages of prescribed medications, while staying on top of the worst symptoms of the conditions. There is ample space given to the issue of the side effects caused by steroid treatment, as this is one of the questions that most bothers people who are living with PMR and GCA. Alternatives to steroids are considered. Readers will notice that alternative therapies do not get much of a look-in in this book. There are two reasons for this. The first is that I have tried to be true both to my own experience and to what scientific evidence I have been able to glean. After eight years of living with PMR and studying it, and confronting the real dangers of not treating GCA, I am, regrettably, convinced that alternative therapies do not have a great deal to offer the treatment of PMR and GCA, especially in the acute phase. I have not been able to find independent, unbiased evidence that alternative therapies work here. We may hate the drugs, but in this case we need them. Sorry.

Chapter 5 tackles the challenge of living with GCA or PMR, once the initial shock of diagnosis has passed, and you have to face the reality of having a long-term debilitating and potentially painful condition. Managing pain can take up a lot of our time and energy. Many people are of working age and have to keep working if they possibly can. Others may have to face the dreadful consequences of their livelihoods being affected negatively, not just now but for the rest of their lives, if their pensions are also going to be reduced by lower earnings while unwell. Through all of this, we have to try to keep active and have some quality of life. This means reassessing how we spend our time, and how much we can give of ourselves to others. For people who are also carers, living with PMR and/or GCA presents particular struggles and dilemmas. Many people are determined to do the very best they can to get themselves better, whatever it takes, and so there is a lot of interest in alternative therapies and how we can modify our diets.

For several years, I have thought that looking at PMR and GCA just as rheumatic conditions is to some extent missing the point. We have to look closer, and look deeper, at what is happening inside our bodies. These are 'auto-immune' conditions. The inflammation that causes our pain is not due to wear and tear, nor to trauma or to injury, but is caused by the normally healthy processes of the immune system. When the immune system gets out of control and goes into overdrive, we suffer conditions linked to chronic inflammation. Autoimmune illnesses can affect the muscles and joints, or the skin and connective tissue, or the gastric system. Perhaps to some extent it is a lottery which of these illnesses we fall prey to. Perhaps we could count ourselves lucky that we 'only' get GCA or PMR. There is no smoke without fire, so having one autoimmune illness is probably an indicator that there might be others lurking around the corner. I have a nice collection to keep me busy into my old age. So Chapter 6 is dedicated to finding out more about autoimmune conditions, what is going on in the body when we have one, and what we can do about it.

In Chapter 7, it's 'let's roll up our sleeves and get on with it' time. You need, while you are reading this book and through the course of your journey with GCA and PMR, to keep repeating the mantra *I am getting better*. Honestly, the chances are that you *will* make a good recovery, however remote that prospect might seem at times. We need to learn to take the long view and believe in our power to heal ourselves. Because that is what we are doing. We can make it easier or harder for ourselves, and this part of the book is about making it easier.

Information about what is happening to change the situation, in the shape of support, awareness and research, is the subject of Chapter 7. How shocking is it that in this day and age, as many as 1000 people a year in the UK can be going completely blind because of a headache? I am writing at the beginning of 2014, when health services in England, where I live, are undergoing a huge change in the way they are delivered. This offers both a challenge and an opportunity. The opportunity for us is to seize the moment and make sight loss through undiagnosed GCA, or late commencement of treatment, a thing of the past.

I've discovered in recent years that people who have PMR and GCA are really interested in research. This shows the hugely generous spirit of people everywhere, because they know that, should there be a great breakthrough, it may come too late for them. So many I have spoken with have said that they want things to be better for people in the future. The bad news is that for many years, PMR and GCA have been research backwaters, not where researching doctors would want to go in order to make a name for themselves, and not where pharmaceutical companies could predict good returns. One expert on PMR told me that for every one research project on PMR, there are ten on rheumatoid arthritis.

The good news is that things are beginning to change, and there is a groundswell of interest and activity. I believe we are on the verge of a major breakthrough. As a trustee of PMRGCAuk, a charity dedicated to providing support, raising awareness, and fostering research, I am very committed to this organisation's success, and proceeds from the publication of this book will be donated to the charity. I would like to stress though that all the opinions expressed in this work, and any mistakes in it, are my own, and not the responsibility of PMRGCAuk. In order to make the book as readable as possible, I have not used academic conventions with numerous references and footnotes. However, the information I present is backed up with reference to published sources listed in the References section. If you have any queries please contact me.

The book is written from the perspective of a UK-based

former patient involved with a UK charity. All my personal experience has been in the English NHS system. Some of the clinical information included may be based on assumptions, e.g. about health service structures and prescribing practices, that are different in other countries. I apologise for this shortcoming (though not for the British English spellings!) and hope that readers in other countries will still find the book helpful and supportive.

It is now more than four years since I last took a steroid pill. For a long time I kept a bubble pack of 5mg tabs in my bedside drawer just in case. I am confident now that the PMR really has left me. So much so that I am even beginning to forget what that pain and stiffness felt like. I hope that before too long, you will have the same feeling that you have at last slain the dragon of PMR or GCA.

2: POLYMYALGIA RHEUMATICA

What is Polymyalgia Rheumatica?

Literally translated, the term *'polymyalgia rheumatica'* means 'muscle pain all over the place', which tells us a bit about the symptoms but very little about what the illness actually is.

The British Society for Rheumatology and the British Health Professionals in Rheumatology publish guidelines for the management of PMR. These state: "PMR is the most common inflammatory rheumatic disease in the elderly and is one of the biggest indications for long-term steroid therapy. There are difficulties in diagnosis, with heterogeneity in presentation, response to steroids and disease course." This is actually the closest these guidelines get to a definition. The use of the term 'elderly' is interesting, and controversial. It is true that the average age of onset is about 72. But that is an average. PMR actually strikes people over the age of 50, being very rare among people under the age of 50. People in their fifties do not consider themselves elderly, and the use of the word, I think, tends to create a stereotype in the minds of many clinicians about what the 'typical' patient is like. I also suspect that it has an effect on how 'interesting' PMR is seen to be among doctors. These guidelines are, at the time of writing, being revised, and representatives of patient groups have made a strong argument that the word 'elderly' should be dropped in favour of 'older people'.

A paper by Dahiya and Hazleman (2005), published in a journal of geriatric medicine, describes PMR as an "inflammatory condition of unknown aetiology [meaning causation]... It is a clinical syndrome characterised by aching and stiffness in the neck, shoulders, and pelvic girdles [sic], systemic symptoms and a raised erythrocyte sedimentation rate (ESR). It usually responds rapidly to low doses of corticosteroid and has a favourable prognosis."

This is getting us a little closer to a definition, with a focus on pain and stiffness, but it still admits that the cause is unknown. Medical consensus now more or less agrees that PMR is an autoimmune inflammatory illness, meaning that the autoimmune system has become overactive and out of control, creating excessive inflammation in various parts of the body.

Now, your doctor may have told you that PMR is a condition of the muscles. Certainly, if you have PMR you feel intense pain in your muscles, perhaps in your shoulders or the tops of your arms. However, there is little, if any, evidence from studies that the muscles themselves are diseased. The problem seems to lie somewhere else. The overlap with Giant Cell Arteritis seems to suggest that it lies in the circulation system, as a form of vasculitis caused by a dysfunction of the autoimmune system.

There will be more information about autoimmune illness in Chapter 4. In this chapter, we will look more closely at the ways in which medical science is trying to cast light on the mystery of PMR and improve approaches to diagnosis and treatment.

The PMR classification study

The PMR classification study, carried out by the American College of Rheumatology (ACR) and the European League Against Rheumatism (EULAR), surveyed 111 rheumatologists and 53 non-rheumatologists in North America and Western Europe. The survey was designed to boil down the many and various criteria that clinicians use around the world to a manageable set that everybody could agree on. This meant systematically weeding out those criteria that are peripheral or not sufficiently well represented across *all* cases of PMR. This is tremendously important, because it opens the doors to international research and the possibility of comparing research results across different studies, knowing that everybody is talking about the same thing when they are talking about PMR. The study started with no less than 68 potential criteria, and progressively narrowed them down to seven.

The Magnificent Seven are:

        a.   The person is aged 50 or over

        b.   Symptoms have lasted at least two weeks

    c.   Aching of *both* shoulders and/or pelvic girdle aching (the bilateral aspect is very important)

    d.   Morning stiffness lasting at least 45 minutes

    e.   An elevated erythrocyte sedimentation rate (ESR)

    f.   An elevated C-reactive protein level in the blood (CRP)

    g.   Rapid response to corticosteroids

All of these received unanimous support in Round Two of the study: in other words, all the clinicians and scientists agreed that these should be included as the key classification criteria. It is worth noting one or two of the criteria that did not quite make it. There was a high level of agreement (84%) for including limitation of shoulder movement, and slightly lower agreement (76%) for including restricted hip mobility. 'Peripheral' symptoms such as carpal tunnel syndrome and tenosynovitis were eliminated from the criteria. These also appear in some cases of PMR but not in sufficient numbers to warrant inclusion.

Each of the Magnificent Seven of the classification criteria for PMR merits a closer look.

a. Aged 50 or over

Does this mean that if you are younger than 50 you cannot have PMR? Well, not exactly, although it does give an indication of how rare it is in younger people. The average

age of onset of PMR is 72. This leads doctors to believe that it has some kind of connection with the ageing process. I found it very difficult, in my mid-50s, to come to terms with having an illness that elderly people are supposed to get. I hadn't even really got used to thinking of myself as middle-aged. The menopause had been going on and I had been taking HRT. I felt full of beans and pretty fit. However, the fact is that in any distribution curve, there will be people at the extreme ends, the 'outliers' who aren't typical.

For the unlucky few who do get PMR in their early 50s or even earlier, doctors are extremely unwilling to diagnose PMR unless they are quite certain that all other possibilities have been eliminated. It is more likely that an alternative diagnosis would be correct. The reluctance to diagnose is because putting people onto a course of steroids that may last two years or even longer is an extremely serious matter, even when the steroids are the right treatment. In the case of a young person wrongly diagnosed with PMR, the steroids will probably mask the symptoms of something else, potentially more sinister, going on. For this and other reasons, if you are younger than 55 and diagnosed with PMR by your GP, I would strongly recommend that you make a very strong case for a referral to a rheumatology clinic, for the very simple reason that your young age makes you an 'atypical' patient.

b. Symptoms lasting at least two weeks

Sometimes people have been suffering for ages before they go to the doctor, and cannot even remember when it all started. Others have tried all kinds of remedies, or have suffered in silence, believing themselves to be afflicted with 'the aches and pains of growing older'. PMR is much more than that. Doctors have to allow a certain length of time for symptoms to have been happening, in order to rule out symptoms of a fever, such as flu, or an injury, like muscle strain from over-exertion.

c. Aching of both shoulders (bilateral aching) and/or pelvic girdle aching

Like many people, I had long ago got used to aching shoulders. They have been a fact of life ever since office work became computer work. Most of us working in sedentary jobs are familiar with the chronic tension in our shoulders and necks, reaching a crescendo by the end of the day, bringing on the classic 'tension headache' on the journey home. So how is the pain of PMR different from this? My customary shoulder tension and ache was around my shoulder blades. The PMR pain seemed to start right on the ridge of my shoulders and radiate up into my neck and down into my upper arms. Getting dressed, doing up my bra, brushing my hair were particularly painful.

It wasn't until I started to find it really difficult getting up from my office chair that I realised the pain was spreading. I was feeling it deeper in my body, deep down inside the muscles, and almost even deeper than that. I knew at the same time that my actual joints, my shoulder and hip joints that is, the bony bits, were absolutely fine. So much so that it used to irritate me beyond reason when some kind-hearted soul would ask 'And how are your joints today?'

For some PMR sufferers who have the illness particularly severely, the pain is intense, like a Chinese burn, except that you cannot kick your little brother to make it stop. It is more, far more, than feeling a bit achy.

The pain of PMR is felt in *the proximal muscles*. These large muscles do the incredibly important job of connecting the limbs and head to the body, and provide the motor engines for the joints that move our arms, legs and head. They extend from the upper limbs onto the trunk, and are aided and abetted by a complex system of tendons, ligaments, and, of course, arteries, that provide fuel in the form of oxygenated blood. In some people, there is also pain in the hands, in the carpal tunnels. Also, about one in five PMR patients also present at the time of diagnosis with GCA symptoms such as severe headache and visual disturbance.

This leads to the speculative question whether the reason that GCA and PMR seemed to be linked in some way is that PMR is also a form of arteritis. Could this be so? There is a school of thought, it is true, that holds that PMR is a form of vasculitis, or inflammation of the blood vessels, in many cases. We cannot say for sure that *all* cases of PMR are necessarily linked to inflammation in the blood vessels, rather than inflammation in other tissues. However, the idea seems intuitively to make sense. If the big muscles are hurting because they are short of oxygen, then it stands to reason that they will feel awfully stiff and unwilling to move. If only things were that simple!

21

At the first International Symposium on PMR and GCA, held in Chelmsford in 2012, I stood up and asked one eminent researcher "Why, if there is all this evidence that PMR is a form of vasculitis, are patients usually told by their doctor that they have a problem with their muscles, or their joints?" He looked at me with some surprise. "I don't know", came the answer.

We cannot very well open people up and check inside the walls of their arteries. Ultrasound scans offer some promise of 'looking' into and identifying inflammation, but ultrasound is expensive and training ultrasound technicians is a slow process. Like it or not, PMR is unlikely to be very high on the priorities list for ultrasound or other imaging techniques in every rheumatology unit for a long time to come. The temporal artery biopsy for suspected cases of GCA, which takes away a small 'expendable' section of artery from just below the skin of the temple, is the closest we can get to definite evidence of what is going on deep down. Biopsy is not available for PMR, which is a tricky illness that 'mimics' many other conditions.

d. Morning stiffness

Ah, morning stiffness. This one makes me smile, and not in a good way. I felt stiff *all the time*. That phrase 'morning stiffness' often raises a hollow laugh among groups of PMR sufferers. We are probably all familiar with the sensation of waking up feeling as though our limbs and back have turned into MDF during the night. In a healthy person, stretching like a cat will get everything moving again. Not so with polymyalgia rheumatica. People with PMR tell stories of having to be physically manhandled into a sitting position by a long-suffering partner.

There were times, in the early hours of the morning, when I would cry out in pain, half-asleep, and my husband would patiently get out of bed, come round to my side, and turn me over. What must it be like for people on their own? We heard about one woman who tied a rope to rails on the foot of her bed so that she could haul herself up inch by inch like a mountain climber. Other people have taken to sleeping in an armchair (not recommended).

The stiffness is not only present in the morning. A large proportion of PMRGCAuk members report that they experience stiffness *whenever* they have been sitting or standing still for any length of time, at any time of the day. Drivers, on reaching their destination, have to lift their legs up to put them outside the car and plant their feet on the ground. In meetings, we have to get up and walk around to loosen ourselves up. Otherwise, we make an exhibition of ourselves when the meeting ends. Asking for a push-up from a colleague can be a bit embarrassing, and not very dignified.

While doctors tend to make a clear distinction between pain and stiffness, for PMR sufferers they are two sides of the same coin. They are the evil twins that stalk us, always together. The pain is associated with rigidity, and the stiffness – well, it bloody well hurts. It is not like the almost pleasant stiffness and ache that comes into tired muscles after some intense physical activity, like walking up a mountain, or doing a day's gardening. It is miserable and debilitating. It is not the kind of stiffness that melts away with a warm bath or a good massage. If only it did! I used to be a great fan of a strong Swedish massage before I got PMR. While I had PMR, I would not have been able to tolerate such firm pressure on my shoulders.

e. Elevated ESR

The ESR (Erythrocyte Sedimentation Rate) test is a blood test that measures the rate at which red blood cells settle in a blood sample within a period of one hour. *Erythrocyte* is the scientific term for a red blood cell. The rate of sedimentation of these cells in a sample of anti-coagulated blood is an indicator of inflammation of the body. A substance called fibrinogen, also present in the blood, increases in quantity when there is inflammation present, and this causes the red blood cells to stick together, becoming heavier and falling to the bottom of the tube. Thus, a higher sedimentation rate is a general indicator of inflammation. However, it is a bit of a blunt instrument. While a 'normal' ESR level in a healthy middle-aged adult might be around 20 to 22, a person with PMR or GCA might have a rate over 100. Yet if the ESR returns to normal, or towards normal, it does not necessarily mean that there is no disease present. Throughout my illness, my ESR rate never went above 50 (for this reason I was classified as 'atypical') and most of the time it was around 28 while I was on steroids. However, I was evidently and obviously ill. Another limitation of the ESR test is that it has to be carried out within four hours of the blood being taken.

f. Elevated CRP

Cytokines are protein molecules secreted by various organs in the body and are part of the system by which cells communicate with each other. One category of cytokine in the interleukin (IL-1, IL-6 and so on). IL-6 is a little number that is released to stimulate the immune response. As it is the immune system going into battle that triggers inflammation in various parts of the body, the levels of IL-6 are a good indication of the levels of inflammation. C-Reactive Protein (CRP) is a substance that interacts with IL-6 and plays a part in cleaning up the molecular debris caused by cell death and breakdown. Its level rises rapidly in phases of acute inflammation, sometimes as much as 50,000-fold. It follows that the C-Reactive Protein test is a haematological (blood) test that gives a measure of, yes, you guessed it, inflammation in the body. Researchers have found that levels of IL-6 and CRP are far higher in people with PMR than with late onset rheumatoid arthritis, and this is one of the ways of distinguishing these two conditions. Tests to measure IL-6 are expensive, but the CRP test is relatively cheap.

The biochemistry of all these reactions and counter-reactions going on, triggered by and modified by the immune system, is incredibly complicated and finely balanced. It is not surprising if in some individuals, these tests turn out not to be terribly reliable when it comes to judging how a patient with a disease such as PMR or GCA is progressing.

g. Rapid response to steroids

You should feel remarkably better, sometimes within hours. About a 70% improvement in symptoms should be felt within a week, at the longest. That is, you should be able to say that 70% of your pain and stiffness is relieved. However, GPs should not use the response to steroids to diagnose PMR. This is because almost any inflammatory illness will respond in the short term to steroids. PMR means putting people on them for a couple of years or more, and is not something to be taken lightly, or in a spirit of 'let's suck it and see'. For a doctor to take the line 'I'll put you on the steroids and we'll see what happens', would be irresponsible, because the dose could mask all sorts of other illnesses. Before the patient is put onto steroids, many other possibilities need to be ruled out, such as rheumatoid arthritis, and various cancers. The reaction to steroids should also be *sustained* over time. If they seem to 'stop working' after a short while, this might call the initial diagnosis of PMR into question.

Diagnosis of PMR – to refer or not to refer

We can see that PMR is tricky to diagnose. It is largely a process of eliminating everything else. PMR is what you are left with, and a diagnosis of PMR will be supported by high ESR and CRP values in blood tests. A recent study has indicated that up to half of the cases thought by GPs to be PMR are not PMR at all. This means that thousands of people may be on long-term steroid medication who do not need to be. Thus, although PMR is not really a life-threatening illness, there are many reasons why we need to improve diagnosis. This raises the question whether PMR should be treated in primary care, by general practitioners, or be referred to consultant rheumatologists.

GPs tend to refer only the 'atypical' or tricky cases to consultant rheumatologists at the local hospital. This means that rheumatologists do not get to see the majority of 'typical' cases and they do not get to include these cases in their research studies. One consequence of this is that research into PMR might be skewed by having an unrepresentative sample. PMR is an under-researched illness. If all suspected cases were referred, specialists would soon appreciate the extent of the problem and it might, just might, attract more research attention.

Putting anybody onto long-term steroid treatment carries risks to their health, and so it could be argued that everyone with suspected PMR should be referred to a specialist for assessment. However, it is unlikely that there will be a recommendation in guidelines for all cases of polymyalgia rheumatica to be referred at the time of diagnosis. Referral would be appropriate if an alternative to prednisolone might be a better option for people with complex pre-existing conditions, or certain risk factors complicate the prognosis. There are other social and economic factors that I refer to below, that might also justify referral. Another issue in diagnosis is that many rheumatologists consider that PMR is being over-diagnosed by family doctors. One study in Bristol, in which GPs agreed to refer *all* diagnosed cases of PMR to the rheumatology clinic, found that 50% of the patients did not have PMR at all. And that means that many people must be being put onto long-term steroids inappropriately.

Here is the story of Val's experience of being diagnosed, or not diagnosed, with PMR. It is a particularly messy case, but by no means unusual. I reproduce Val's story in her own words here just to give a flavour of how confusing and distressing it can be. I am not going to make any comment: you can draw your own conclusions.

Val's story

I am 72yrs old... About a year ago, I was having pains in my shoulders and arms, and stiffness in my shoulders. Getting out of bed in the morning was torture as I was in so much pain that it made me cry with every move. It felt like flu but I knew it wasn't. So I went to see the GP who said, "I am almost 99% sure that you have PMR but I would like you to see a rheumatologist as I do not want to start you on steroids until we have a more concrete result."

I had to wait a couple of months before I got an appointment, and was taking Cocodamol for the pain. The rheumatologist said that she was not sure if it was PMR or Fibromyalgia and she would take some blood tests etc. She then told me that as she was retiring she would make an appointment for me to see the rheumatologist that was taking over from her, but this lady would not be able to see me for another six months, and in the interim I should take pain killers.

I went back to my GP and asked her if perhaps I could have a second opinion, and she agreed, and asked if I had anyone in mind. I said that there was a neurologist in another hospital, and could I see her if possible? GP agreed, and an appointment came through very soon after.

This Neurologist was extremely nice, and she said that I do not have Neurology problems, but my ESR level was 32/33 and this was rated as being high. (This consultation was in June of last year, and a couple of weeks later, I was asked to go to see my GP who told me that the Neurologist had confirmed that I do have PMR and that I should be taking steroids and that I should be monitored on a regular basis. Soon after seeing my GP the GP told me that she was going to be on Maternity leave until end of Feb this year, and one of the other doctors would take care of me....

After a few hours of taking the Preds, I was actually started in 20mg per day. The pain disappeared and I became like a spring chicken, all stiffness gone. This other doctor did monitor me every 2 weeks for about 2 months, then he said that I should be thinking of reducing the Preds, in order to come off them as soon as possible...., from 20mg to 18, then 16/then 15, and for the past 4/5/ weeks 12.5 & 12mg. The GP said that being on them since 19th July 2013 was a long ɔ̣̃e

*ᶦot sure if I really had PMR and because of
  ᴜe simply aches and pains as this is what
  ᴜple get, and the only way was to take pain killers.
ᴧot being happy with this, I went to see one of the other
doctors in the surgery, and she told me that perhaps I should
see a rheumatologist at the local hospital, as the neurologist
had discharged me for my own GP to be looking after me as
we had the diagnosis.*

*Before taking the Pred, I was unable to lift my arms, this
went when I started them, now I am finding it difficult to lift
them again, I have been putting it down to the reduction of
the Pred.*

*When this rheumatologist told me that in his opinion I did
not have PMR he said, "You do not get pain with it",
although he prodded me on the shoulders and arms. He said
with PMR you definitely do not get pain....He said he was
also not sure but it could be Fibromyalgia but again not so
sure about that either. He told me to have some more blood
tests taken and would see me again in May, I said if what
you are telling me, that I am going to be in extreme pain,
and finding that paracetamol does not work, could he
recommend something else, his response was "go to a pain
clinic, I don't deal with pain."*

So this is where we are up to.

Early treatment of PMR

The British Society of Rheumatologists guidelines for the treatment of PMR suggest starting the patient off on 15mg of prednisolone per day, with a progressive tapering down once symptoms have been stabilized. As we have noted already, the glucocorticosteroid prednisolone is the drug of choice for PMR. It works, in that it deals with the symptoms and restores something approaching normal life to the patient. It is an unusually cheap drug as well, which is fortunate for the NHS, but perhaps not so fortunate for the PMR patient. If a prednisolone tablet costs 2p, then the prednisolone for somebody who starts on 15mg per day and tapers down to nothing after two years, is going to cost the NHS the princely sum of £30. It is no wonder that prednisolone is the drug of choice for PMR. It does the job. It removes the worst of the pain. It restores quality of life and it keeps people out of the doctor's surgery. And it is cheap as chips.

Although I do not have any concrete evidence for this, only 'gut feeling' after listening to many patients' stories, my view is that many (not all) doctors regard PMR as an old women's illness. Elderly women in western society are generally discounted, joked about, and rendered invisible in public life. They tend to be stereotyped, and this stereotyping needs to be countered. PMR patients should be assessed not only on their physical condition, but also consulted with about social and circumstantial factors such as the following:

a. Is this patient a man or a woman? Bearing in mind that often men will be averse to admitting they are having a difficult time of it.

b. Is this person in employment? What is the nature of their employment and how sympathetic/supportive is their employer likely to be?

c. Is this person in their 50s (or even late 40s)? In my view, *every* case under 55 should be referred to a specialist rather than being treated solely in primary care. I regard very young age as a 'complicating factor'.

d. Is this person a carer? If they were unable to continue caring because of PMR/GCA, what would the consequences be for the family?

e. What is their current level of physical activity? How can they be helped to continue their physical activity, maybe at a reduced level? Would physiotherapy be of any help? (should routinely be asked at various stages in the course of the illness)

f. Does this person already have weight/obesity issues? How can this person best be helped to maintain and if possible improve their nutrition while they have PMR?

g. How proactive is this person likely to be in managing their condition themselves? How can

they best be encouraged to access sources of
information and support that will be able to help
them? Who else in their lives needs to know about
and understand PMR?

A GP should include such social and personal factors in the
assessment of whether or not a case needs to be referred
to a rheumatology clinic. Granted, PMR is generally not life
threatening and people who start well have a fair prospect
of recovery, but it is a serious illness and potentially grave
because of the collateral damage it can do. I am not
suggesting that doctors should take all the burden of this on
themselves, but at least have the conversation that treats
the patient holistically and as an individual. Also informing
all patients of the risk and cardinal symptoms of GCA is
paramount. It is amazing how many PMR patients have no
idea. It is as though, having finally got a diagnosis, the GP
breathes a sigh of relief, writes the script, and shows the
patient the door.

The PMRGCAuk helpline regularly takes calls from people
newly diagnosed with PMR who are struggling to come to
terms with the diagnosis and what it means for them. It is
striking that the most common concern voiced by these
'new' patients is the fear of being 'on steroids' for a long
time. Some are worried that their starting dose is so high,
and have not understood that it will drop over time. Many
people want to avoid starting on them altogether and are
looking for a viable alternative. They ask whether they can
'manage' without taking the steroids, and whether, say,
paracetamol might be an adequate substitute.

Many patients are anxious about the side effects they have heard about, particularly the 'moon face' (otherwise known as Cushing syndrome), weight gain, and alterations to the skin and hair growth. This anxiety is justified and perfectly understandable. However, the difficult truth is that the consequences of not taking the steroids, for most people, carry more risks than taking them. To begin with, there is the risk that PMR, if left untreated, might develop into Giant Cell Arteritis, for those patients whose vascular system is also implicated in their PMR. Secondly, and just as serious, is the effect that PMR has on daily life, and the quality of life. Most people simply cannot manage daily life with PMR without the medication. We are talking about an illness that literally makes it impossible for people to get themselves out of bed in the morning. Dressing, self-care, even going to the toilet, become major feats of endurance.

When I started taking the steroids, within hours I went from hobbling with a walking stick to running up the stairs. It felt like a miracle. It was a miracle. People who have not experienced PMR might find it difficult to understand what 'muscle pain all over the place' really is like. For me the stiffness was of a completely different order from any kind of stiffness I had ever experienced before, including the stiffness after running the London marathon. Then, if I mustered all my will, I could make my body move. The stiffness of PMR was more like a paralysis. However much I talked to my body and teased it, entreated it, implored it to move, it would not. The pain went beyond any pain I had ever experienced in my muscles or joints before. With this level of pain, it is impossible to concentrate, to work, to get on with daily life. PMR makes people literally *dis*-abled. The steroids give us our lives back. But at a cost. Chapter 3 takes a closer look at what that cost might be.

Your doctor may direct you to take all your tablets at once, early in the day. This is for two reasons. Firstly because your symptoms may very well be worse in the mornings, and secondly because prednisolone may have the effect of keeping you awake if taken at night. Your doctor may instruct you to follow a low salt, high potassium, or high calcium diet. Your doctor will probably also prescribe or recommend a calcium or potassium supplement, to protect bone density. Follow these directions carefully and if possible, get a bone scan.

Talk to your doctor about eating grapefruit and drinking grapefruit juice while you are taking this medication. However, the effect of grapefruit juice on the interaction of prednisolone with your body is not thought to be as great as with some other drugs. So it may be that you can still enjoy a glass of grapefruit juice with your breakfast without causing any serious problems.

Issues in the diagnosis and treatment of PMR

As we have seen, there seems to be little doubt now that PMR, like GCA, is connected to the circulation system and is probably some form of vasculitis, or inflammation in the lining of the blood vessels (as well as other places such as the *bursas,* the sacs of fluid surrounding the shoulder joints).

Could it be that the more severe cases or cases where there are repeated relapses are the ones that would show up as having, or leading to, large vessel vasculitis? PET scans seem to indicate that the long-sought 'missing link' between GCA and PMR might be large vessel vasculitis, affecting in particular the subclavian arteries near the shoulders. One study found that over 50% of new GCA patients also had large vessel inflammation elsewhere in the body. So could it be possible that *all* cases of PMR have some kind of vascular involvement? At the moment, it is not possible to be sure, but the suspicion is there. Here I am speculating, but I have discussed this with several experts and none of them has contradicted me.

This is important for us as patients, because it suggests that we really must take good care of our circulation systems, eating a healthy diet low in salt, saturated fat and refined carbohydrates (sugars and starches). And we need to do this for life.

At the 2012 International Symposium on PMR and GCA, Professor Marco Cimmino gave a rundown of work on new treatments. According to his figures, 38% of patients have at least one recurrence, with 25% suffering from repeated relapses. These are the people who would benefit most from effective new treatments because at the moment their doses of steroids are 'yo-yo-ing' up and down. A recently developed nighttime release form of prednisolone is proving very helpful for some patients, because the level of

IL-6, the blood chemical that is the big culprit in our inflammation and pain, is at its highest in the small hours of the morning. For this reason, Cimmino and others suggest that not everybody is best taking all their prednisolone first thing in the morning. If you are having problems reducing your steroid dose, or you feel particularly unwell first thing in the morning, you might discuss with your doctor the possibility of taking some of it in the evening, so that it is in your system in the small hours, when the levels of IL-6 are highest. If this does not suit you, you could try waking up early and taking the steroids an hour or so before you need to get up, in order to let them settle into your body and start working before you have to get moving.

Prednisolone is so cheap and so effective in suppressing inflammation in straightforward cases, that it is unlikely it will be abandoned in favour of more expensive drugs such as the new generation of 'biologics'. However, there is a lot of interest in 'steroid sparing' because consultants are deeply concerned about the damaging effects of steroids on the body (even though they might not show it to you!). A new drug called Tocilizumab is showing great potential in cases of rheumatoid arthritis, and is being trialled for GCA (although not for PMR). Results may show that it might work without steroids. Methotrexate (MTX) has mixed results in research, but latest findings suggest that it may be most effective in those cases that also have large vessel vasculitis. In the UK, rheumatologists are only likely to prescribe MTX in complex cases. In other countries, Poland, for example, its use for PMR is routine. There is a new prednisolone formulation in combination with a drug called dipyridamole, which, it is claimed, makes the prednisolone ten times as effective as it is by itself but this is not yet being used for PMR.

One study has demonstrated that being of lower weight is an indicator of better results with steroids. One European specialist is calculating starting dose at 0.2mg per day for each kilogram of the patient's weight. Thus, a small patient weighing only 50kg would start on 10mg per day, and a large person of 100kg or more would start on 20mg per day. This makes sense. At the time of writing, the international PMR guidelines group is still discussing what to say in terms of initial dosage, because practice is different from country to country.

Starting people off on high doses of prednisolone increases the possibility of diagnostic error, because almost anything will respond to high dose steroids. The patient needs to be assessed for rapid, sustained, and more or less complete response (defined as 70% improvement in pain and stiffness symptoms).

Prof Christian Mallen, of Keele University, is leading a team carrying out research into the primary care diagnosis and early treatment of PMR. Christian points out that most research data comes from people who have been referred to rheumatology departments, and as these are often 'atypical' cases, it is important to do research on patients in primary care, who represent a more 'typical' population. The Keele team have found that PMR patients are more likely than other patients in the same age group to go to their GP with fatigue symptoms *before* they are diagnosed, and more likely to present with anxiety *after* diagnosis. He suggests that PMR patients need time to discuss their worries, especially about steroid treatment.

Have I got GCA?

When I was diagnosed with polymyalgia rheumatica I was not told about Giant Cell Arteritis, and a survey by PMRGCAuk patients revealed that a majority of new PMR patients have the same experience. I believe that *everyone* diagnosed with PMR should be warned to watch out for the cardinal symptoms of GCA, namely:

1. Sudden onset severe headache, usually on one side

2. Tender scalp

3. Tenderness of the temple region, possibly with visible swelling of the artery

4. Jaw claudication on chewing (sometimes talking)

5. Blurred or interrupted vision.

Around 20-25% of people with PMR also have GCA at the same time. GCA of course is the more acute problem and so these patients will be on a higher dose of steroids. Then there is a small proportion of people who develop GCA later, often after they have had PMR for some time and their steroid dose has been tapered down. A flare-up of PMR may be accompanied by the arrival of GCA.

Even without the appearance of 'full-blown' GCA, many PMR patients report a range of symptoms that have been described by some clinicians as 'sub-clinical' GCA symptoms. Headaches, sometimes quite serious, feverishness, blurriness of the vision, lasting for a few minutes to a few hours. This can be very alarming and create anxiety that these symptoms are about to escalate into 'full-blown' GCA. How worried should you be if this happens to you?

If the symptom is just blurriness on its own, it may not be so much the PMR itself as some other inflammation going along with the PMR. What I mean is that, because PMR is an autoimmune inflammatory illness, there is every reason why you might have autoimmune inflammation going on somewhere else as well. For example, inflammation of the eyelids is called *blepharitis*, and it can cause blurry vision especially when your eyes are tired.

Steroid therapy, especially at the higher doses, can also provoke blurry vision. This is because the steroids increase the amount of glucose in your blood and other bodily fluids. Your body tries to compensate by retaining fluid to bring the balance back to normal. This fluid retention or build-up can alter the normal curvature of your eye and have an impact on the quality of your vision. This effect is usually temporary though and rights itself. It is, however, quite unpleasant at the time.

I had laser surgery for long sight when I was coming off the steroids. I had been very long-sighted since birth, and my glasses had got progressively thicker and thicker until they were the proverbial bottle ends. As a child, when I dreamed about a fairy godmother offering me a wish, it was always to be able to chuck the glasses away. So when I realised that laser was at last available for long sight, I set about finding somebody to fix my eyes. One surgeon refused to do it while I had PMR because he predicted I would have an inflammatory reaction. But another surgeon agreed to do it and guess what? I had an inflammatory reaction! Nevertheless, through the experience I also learned a lot about eyes, eyelids and tears.

Our tears are made up of three layers that are secreted by different sets of glands. The meibomian glands in our eyelids make an oily layer that sits on top of the watery tears and prevents them evaporating. If this layer is not working for some reason, for instance because of blepharitis, our eyes get dry, although paradoxically they may feel teary because our other glands are churning out tears to make up for the evaporation. There are simple steps we can take to control dry eye.

Warmth can be very effective. Try doing this at night. Soak a clean face cloth in very hot water. Wring it out, fold it and lay it over your eyes. It is surprisingly comforting. As it cools down put it in the water again to heat it up. Do this treatment for about ten minutes. This will help unblock the glands. Every couple of days, in the morning, dilute a couple of drops of Johnson's baby shampoo on a cotton pad or facecloth and use this to clean along the edge of your eyelids. Don't worry, it won't sting! You can be quite vigorous, sweeping the pad along your eyelashes and massaging the eyelids at the same time. This will clean away any debris like dead skin cells and make your eyelids as clean as - well, as clean as anything. After a few days of this, you may find that things are a lot better. If not, get yourself a bottle of eyedrops (intensive for dry eyes) from Boots and use them about four times a day. If none of this works, then tell the doctor. I paid the price of a small secondhand car for this information and I'm telling you for nothing!

Occasionally things are more serious and GCA may appear in a minority of cases. For me, this is one of the clearest indications that PMR and GCA are both manifestations of vascular disease. Everyone with PMR should know the symptoms of GCA and be vigilant about following up symptoms. The awareness of this link should also help us to counter any suggestion, either from our doctors, or from those near to us, that our aches and pains are just a 'normal' part of growing older. They are not. The aches and pains and feverishness of PMR are signs of a serious, systemic illness, one that affects our whole bodies. The *disease* of PMR may be felt in the large muscles, but it is not restricted to them.

3: GIANT CELL ARTERITIS

What is Giant Cell Arteritis?

If you are going to be ill with something for two years, you might as well know how to pronounce it properly. We have all heard of arthritis, but few people outside medicine have ever heard of *art-er-it is*. The *'-itis'* bit of the word means 'inflammation'. In the case of GCA, we are talking about 'inflammation of the arteries', not *arthritis,* which means 'inflammation of the joints'. People often get these two words mixed up. To be honest, GPs are not very good at checking out with patients whether they have actually understood the name of their illness. It is even more confusing because, surprisingly, this illness falls into the category of rheumatoid or musculoskeletal illness, rather than the category of vascular illness, or illness of the blood circulation system. The specialist you are most likely to see is a rheumatologist rather than a specialist in the circulation system. Don't rheumatologists deal with rheumatoid arthritis? Yes! So just remember that this is art-*er*-it is, and tell all your family and friends how to pronounce it, explain that it means inflammation of the arteries, and instruct them on no account ever to ask you 'how's your arthritis?'.

What actually happens in GCA is that strange giant cells

form in the inner wall of the artery. These cells, compared with normal cells, really are giants. It is like comparing a child's birthday balloon with a hot air balloon in the sky. Those of us born during or just after World War II will remember seeing barrage balloons hanging in the sky. Compared with a normal healthy cell, a giant cell looks like a barrage balloon compared with a child's. Nobody knows for sure what causes these cells to form. They accumulate in the inner membrane, or *lumen,* of the arteries that feed blood to all parts of the head.

The danger is that these giant cells can narrow the inner channel of the artery and cut off the blood supply to key parts of the body, particularly the eyes. Generally, because there is a good network of blood vessels into the head, the blood tries to find a way through that is not blocked, and so all the parts of the head – brain, ears, mouth, nose and the eyes, can get an adequate supply. This is why people will often notice other symptoms before noticing any serious interference with their vision.

Probably the most common symptom of Giant Cell Arteritis is pain somewhere in the head, a signal of blockage. This pain can be acute and throbbing. There are many more common causes of pain in the head, as we all know. Infection, such as a cold or flu, bright sunlight, stress, a cricked neck or too much wine the night before, can all trigger a nasty headache. Other rare conditions can present very much like GCA, and this might be a clue as to why younger people (in their 40s) are sometimes initially suspected of having GCA. One such condition is 'crowned dens syndrome', when crystals form in the 'dens', which in layperson's terms is the hollow in the upper vertebra that the skull balances in. Ouch!

The headache of GCA is usually on one side only, at least at first, and is particularly severe. One sufferer described it as wanting to put her head in a bucket of iced water. However, it is not always as severe as that, and sometimes the headache is absent altogether.

So what other symptoms are there? Occasionally, having a very tender scalp is a sign. One patient has described how trying to brush her hair became excruciatingly painful. Others have spoken of an unbearable tenderness on going to bed, as soon as their head touched the pillow. Pains in the neck may be associated with GCA. Another cardinal symptom is pain in the jaw when chewing. When the supply of oxygenated blood is seriously blocked, the part of the body that is starved of oxygen starts to notice that the oxygen supply is running short. Our tissues need constant oxygen to function, so when they are running short they start to complain to make us take notice. They do this by sending out pain signals. They hurt. This jaw pain is called *claudication (*which means *limping,* because the most common site for claudication is the lower leg). The word goes back to ancient Rome, when the Emperor Claudius had a limp.

The pain in the jaw starts when you start to eat, because the tissues are demanding more fuel to enable them to work harder. Sometimes the pain is so severe that it makes eating solids completely impossible. The pain can sometimes also be felt in the tongue. It subsides when you stop eating. This is an important detail, because it helps to differentiate this claudication from other things that might be causing pain in the jaw, like bone trouble, or an ill-fitting denture.

GCA and vision loss

Things really start to look bad (literally) when visual disturbance comes into the picture. You might experience general fuzziness, blurring, or double vision, and occasionally the sight of one eye might 'go' altogether for a little while and then come back, intermittently. This is the cardinal danger sign for GCA and is a signal to you to get immediate medical help, by going to A and E if necessary. If the blood supply to the optic nerve is cut off altogether, the worst thing that can happen is Anterior Ischaemic Optic Neuropathy (AION), which is effectively a stroke in the eye. The vision damage caused by AION can be total, and is irreversible. This blindness can come on gradually, over a number of days, or happen in just a few hours. In every case it is a medical emergency and every case of suspected GCA should receive immediate treatment to prevent this happening.

There are only 10,000 new cases of GCA a year in the UK. Well, it sounds a lot, but compared with the overall population it is not. It is a good deal rarer than many of the conditions that affect older people. The shocking fact is that, in at least 25% of cases, GCA is only diagnosed after the patient has lost all or some of their sight. This is 2500 cases a year of people's vision being irrevocably damaged by something that is, at least in theory, completely preventable. The Department of Health has accepted the figure of around 3000 people a year losing some of their sight, such as vision loss in one eye. Moreover, up to 1000 of these people are going completely blind, losing their vision in both eyes. We actually do not know the precise numbers. At the time of writing, these figures are extrapolated from local studies. There seems little doubt that Giant Cell, or Temporal Arteritis could be the commonest cause of sudden acute blindness in older people.

This is a truly shocking state of affairs, for a number of reasons. Everyone wants to stay as independent as possible in later life. Younger able-bodied people may not think too much about it, but for the older generation independence is a key aspect of quality of life. Being able to see, to read, use the computer, look after your things, get around, is essential for that independence. Sight becomes the most precious sense as people get older. We realise the penalties of losing our vision, and the gradual deterioration of eyesight that comes with the advancing years becomes a source of anxiety and distress, even to the most active and healthy person. It might be tempting to think that losing one eye is not such a terrible thing. Surely, we might think, we have another to rely on? The reality is more complex. We are designed, like other animals, to have two eyes. They work together. So losing one completely, while the other one has deteriorated, perhaps through glaucoma or macular degeneration, is devastating.

Driving becomes next to impossible with only one eye. You have to relearn how to do everything, and negotiating pavements, kerbs, stairs and even the kitchen, becomes a major challenge.

One woman on the PMRGCAuk helpline talked about the impact that losing the sight in one eye had on her life. She was in her 60s, and was the carer of her older husband, who had a severe life-threatening illness. She had been driving him frequently from their home in the country to his outpatient appointments. This was now impossible for her, since she had lost one eye to GCA, and so they were now both housebound unless they called a taxi, at enormous cost. She was dreading the day he would have to go into hospital, as she would be unable to see him every day. With just one working eye, she found everything difficult to adapt to. Using the telephone, the TV remote control, cooking and shopping, all became more difficult by vision being one-sided. And yet, for her husband's sake, she had to remain cheerful and put a brave face in it.

Another woman who had lost the sight in her right eye had been working as a college lecturer in the north Midlands before she became ill. Living in the countryside, a single parent in her early 50s with a teenage son, she had lost her livelihood because she could no longer drive to work. She and her son were facing a terrible predicament, all because her GP had declared her 'too young' to have GCA.

These stories give the lie to any idea that somehow it does not matter too much if an older person loses their sight. Isn't it just a normal part of getting older? Well, no, it is not. Most people who get GCA would not want to define themselves as old in any case. Most are still active, and many are still working. Many women will be struck with GCA while they are still caring for growing children, or even looking after their own elderly parents. As people are forced to work longer before retirement, we will see more and more working people with polymyalgia rheumatica and giant cell arteritis. Studies suggest that losing sight is one of the worst things that can happen to any human being. One study asked older people how much they valued the sight that they had lost. On average, they reported that they would be prepared to trade a third of their remaining life expectancy to get that sight back. In other words, sight is almost as valuable as life itself. And that was people who had lost the sight in 'only' one eye.

Why are we not making more of a fuss about this? Because if GCA caught in time, the vision loss is completely preventable, with a dose of the glucocorticosteroid drug prednisolone. It is not expensive; it costs just pennies. Prednisolone is one of the cheapest drugs available to the NHS. Once on a daily dose of 60mg of prednisolone, GCA sufferers are protected from vision loss. Those giant cells shrink at the touch of the drug. The inflammation subsides and the blood starts to flow freely again. According to Professor Dasgupta, vision loss from AION never occurs after a person has been on 60mg of prednisolone for five days.

It looks as though a breakthrough has happened in the eye research community, about awareness of GCA and the danger of sight loss. PMRGCAuk forged a new partnership with Fight for Sight, the UK's leading charity funding research to prevent blindness. In June 2013, a small group of members of PMRGCAuk were invited to be part of a one-day workshop, led by the James Lind Alliance, to set the priorities for future research in ophthalmic neuropathy. In lay terms, this means disease of the optic nerve. The 'stroke in the eye' provoked by untreated GCA is technically known as 'anterior ischaemic optic neuropathy', because it irrevocably affects the functioning of the optic nerve.

The workshop involved experts from the College of Ophthalmology, the RNIB, and other leading organisations and patient interest groups. Participants were asked to rank a large number of unanswered questions that had been put forward as candidates to be priorities for research. These ranged from questions about what is actually happening in different parts of the eye at various stages, to 'blue sky' thinking about potential new frontiers such as stem cell research. Through a searching process of discussion, negotiation, head scratching and listening to one another, the long list was eventually whittled down to a 'top 10'. It was exciting to see GCA included several times in the final line-up. Priorities include finding out more about what is actually happening in the optic nerve when anterior ischaemic optic neuropathy occurs, and whether we can ever find a way to make it reversible and restore all or some of the lost sight.

This was a really fascinating day and a learning experience for everybody involved. For the GCA 'representatives', it was a strong indication, perhaps for the first time, that the eye research community is really sitting up and taking notice of the potential disaster of GCA sight loss, which currently is irreversible.

Diagnosis of GCA

Currently there is no absolutely reliable diagnostic instrument for Giant Cell Arteritis, and the best thing we have is the temporal artery biopsy. This is a minor surgical procedure that involves taking a small length of tissue from the artery just under the skin in the temple and examining it to see whether there are any giant cells present. Studies are taking place to find out whether ultrasound might be as effective as biopsy at pinpointing the presence of the giant cells that cause blockage to the arteries carrying blood to the head and eyes. But for now, the biopsy is more reliable than anything else.

Doctors consider that it is important to be 'conservative' in the diagnosis of GCA, i.e. be careful not to diagnose it wrongly, because a positive diagnosis means patients have to go on high doses of steroids for a relatively long period of time. Therefore, it is very important to be able to confirm the diagnosis of GCA. A biopsy of the temporal artery is currently the standard way to do this. A positive biopsy will ideally contain one of the giant cells. For an absolutely confirmed diagnosis, the presence of one or more 'giant cells' will be enough. If the biopsy does not show any evidence of GCA, and the doctor is happy that you do not have GCA, it will be possible to stop the steroid treatment. Unfortunately, though, it does happen rather often that the sample taken does not contain one of these giant cells (perhaps because the sample taken was too short), but the consultant is still confident, because of other symptoms, that the patient actually does have GCA.

It can be quite confusing for the patient, who is feeling unwell anyway so not in the best frame of mind, to discover that, although they have undergone this surgical examination and the biopsy has turned out to be negative, the doctors still are pretty convinced that they have GCA. If that happens to you, you could be forgiven for wondering what the point of the biopsy was in the first place. It is not something to go into lightly, without thinking about it, and without talking things over carefully with your rheumatologist. There is some evidence that the results of the biopsy may give some indication of the severity of the condition. When you are considering whether to have the biopsy, you have to be aware that temporal artery biopsy is not a treatment in itself.

If a rheumatologist recommends a biopsy for your case of suspected GCA, and you agree, you will be asked to sign a consent form prior to your surgery. This involves an explanation of your treatment and any risks involved. By signing this, you agree that an explanation of your treatment and the risks/benefits have been outlined to you in writing and that you agree to the operation.

Before surgery, you can eat, drink and take medications normally. For example, if you normally take warfarin, you do not have to stop taking it. The procedure takes place in the operating theatre. You will need to lie still for 30 to 45 minutes, under local anaesthetic. The surgeon makes an incision in your temple and removes a small section of artery. This is usually only 2cm, or just under an inch, in length. The wound is about 3-4 cm long and, normally, absorbable sutures (stitches) are used. The biopsy then goes for examination under a microscope. You will be able to go home while waiting for the results to come through.

You will have a small dressing to cover the wound on your temple. This stays in place until your follow up appointment, sometimes up to a week later. For a short time, there may be a small amount of pain after the anaesthetic wears off. Taking simple painkillers like paracetamol can help with this. You will need to continue taking the daily steroid dose as advised until your follow up appointment. You can wash your hair carefully.

Every operation, no matter how big or small, carries a possible risk. However, the risks associated with temporal artery biopsy are very small. It is a safe procedure, but the possible complications are:

a. Post-operative infection – look out for redness
    which progressively increases in size, or a
    continuous discharge.

b. Increased inflammation and delayed wound healing
    – temporary redness and swelling to the temple
    area.

c. Bleeding – during the operation and perhaps until
    the evening of procedure. If you are on aspirin or
    warfarin the risk of bleeding is greater.

d. A scar – this is often concealed in the hairline.

Discuss these risks with the rheumatologist and/or the
surgeon before you have the procedure. There are a couple
of serious risks that are fortunately extremely rare.
Temporary or permanent damage to temple region nerves
may produce skin numbness or a drooping brow. Stroke
may result in cases where patient has been diagnosed as
having severe narrowing to the arteries in the neck (carotid
artery disease).

Given that the biopsy is inherently risky, as every operation
is, and a bit of a lottery in terms of whether the giant cell
shows up or not, it is very important that other forms of
diagnostic tool are found. In fact, few patients are informed
that as many as half the biopsy samples taken are useless
because they are not long enough to 'catch' a giant cell. Up

to half of biopsies may be 'false negatives', where the consultant is certain of the GCA diagnosis in spite of the negative biopsy result. In fact, if I knew someone who was facing a biopsy, I would suggest that they ask their consultant the question, "What if the biopsy comes back negative? Will you still think that I have GCA?" The answer to this question might be enough for them to decide whether or not to go ahead with the biopsy.

Let us hope that the TABUL study being carried out in Oxford to test the effectiveness of ultrasound will cast some light on the possibilities. Ultrasound promises to be useful in the identification of GCA and does not involve surgery; the patient can have the test as an outpatient. You might be wondering why ultrasound is not more widely available. One major issue is that ultrasound technicians have to be trained to carry out any procedure, and of course this has to be done by rheumatologists, who are up to their eyes with doing other things. Ultrasound in diagnosis of Giant Cell Arteritis (TABUL) study is being led by Prof. Raashid Luqmani at the Nuffield Orthopaedic Centre in Oxford. This NIHR (National Institute of Health Research) portfolio adopted study has been designed to investigate the specificity and sensitivity of temporal artery biopsy compared to ultrasound for the diagnosis of Giant Cell Arteritis (GCA). The study is funded by the NIHR Health Technology Assessment (HTA, Reference Number HTA Project 08/64/01).

Patients recruited into the study will have an ultrasound scan of the arteries in the side of the head and under the arms, performed before the patient goes for their Temporal Artery Biopsy. The TABUL study will compare the temporal artery ultrasound to temporal artery biopsy, and aims to discover whether ultrasound is as reliable as biopsy, whether it is as acceptable to patients, and whether it is cost effective. The researchers aim to have 430 patients involved in the study. There are around 25-30 hospitals that have signed up to this study. However, recruitment has been slow, one of the reasons being that training of ultrasound clinicians has not happened as quickly in some hospitals as the study's scientific team would have hoped.

Patients can only be recruited into this study when they are first suspected of having GCA, and they must not have had steroids recently for any reason apart from PMR. They will receive an initial clinical assessment, blood tests, ultrasound and biopsy within 7 days of starting high dose steroid treatment. The study includes three visits (baseline, after 2 weeks and at 6 months) and otherwise patients are seen in the normal clinic as required. Further information can be found on:
http://www.ndorms.ox.ac.uk/clinicaltrials.php?trial=tabul

Early treatment of GCA

The standard treatment for GCA is to give the patient high dose glucocorticosteroids, generally *prednisolone,* to control the symptoms. The steroids force the giant cells to shrink and eventually to disappear. Prednisolone is the drug of choice because it works. NSAIDs, or non-steroidal anti-inflammatory drugs, such as ibuprofen, do not have the same effect and you cannot control GCA with them. Currently the recommended starting dose of prednisolone is 60mg per day. Once the symptoms are well under control, doctors will want to start reducing the dose as soon and as quickly as possible.

There is a good deal of debate and speculation about the optimum way of tapering steroids down from this initial high dose. The trick is to reduce the medication as much as possible, since steroids are rather nasty drugs that have other effects on the body, while keeping 'on top of' the symptoms. A patient will hopefully feel very much better very quickly on steroids. However, the illness is still there in the background and reducing the dosage too quickly will result in a flare-up of symptoms. It is important for patients, and doctors too, to understand this and work together in the early weeks to learn how the disease is behaving in the individual, and how the medication is working. Keeping a log of symptoms is a good idea.

If you have been diagnosed with GCA, it is tempting, after the steroids have kicked in and you are feeling much better, hopefully pain free, to think, "OK, that's sorted". The effect of the steroids can literally seem like a miracle. Nevertheless, you need to understand and accept that you have a serious illness. The prednisolone does not cure it – but it does make it possible to live a reasonably normal life, if you are lucky, with GCA.

Issues in the diagnosis and treatment of GCA

Obviously, it is absolutely of the essence that anybody with GCA should be diagnosed and treated as soon as possible. This is easier said than done. As we have already recognised, older people can have headaches for all kinds of reasons. What, though, if vision starts to be disturbed? Imagine that a 76-year old woman called Mary starts to experience blurry vision, as well as headaches. Perhaps she has noticed that her scalp feels tender sometimes. Mary goes to the GP and reports that her sight seems a bit blurry. The doctor is likely to suspect, say, glaucoma, because this is far more common than GCA. If Mary remembers to mention the headaches, the doctor will suggest that Mary goes to the optician, or the ophthalmologist, to have her sight checked out. Meanwhile perhaps she could take paracetamol for the headaches. Probably, Mary completely forgets to mention the occasional tender scalp. Why should she remember it, as it does not seem to have anything to do with the blurriness? She makes an appointment to have her eyes tested. The ophthalmologist, maybe a week or ten days later, checks out her eyes. There may be some signs of glaucoma developing. However, the eye specialist will not see any evidence of the storm that is brewing up in Mary's temporal arteries. Why not? Because the problem is in the arteries, and not in the eyes at all.

Suppose that a man, let us call him Cliff, is experiencing pain in his jaw when he tries to chew his food. His first thought is that his dentures are playing up. Cliff hates going to the dentist, but eventually he plucks up courage. Again, the dentist may not be 'looking in the right place'. It takes a bit of joined-up thinking for a dentist, an ophthalmologist or even a GP to start suspecting GCA.

If a GP does suspect GCA, what should he or she do? GPs report a real dilemma here. The average GP may only see a case of GCA once every three years or so. Some GPs have never seen one. They will ask for blood tests in order to rule out other conditions. Why is it so important for them to do that? Because certain other things that it 'might' be, could actually be life-threatening conditions (like cancer, for example). It is a serious business to put a patient on steroids knowing that they will be on these drugs for two or three years, or even longer. The doctor probably does know that, ideally, Mary or Cliff should be referred to a rheumatologist. If it takes two or three months for the appointment to come through, this may be too late. An alternative is for the GP to start treating the case themselves. The steroids have to be got into those arteries to protect Cliff's or Mary's sight, and the case can't wait for the hospital appointments system to catch up.

All this is very unsatisfactory. A suspected case of GCA now constitutes a 'medical emergency', meaning that the person needs to be seen as soon as possible by a specialist, and probably sent for a biopsy. However, the timescale for dealing with an 'emergency' seems to have become more and more elastic in today's National Health Service. Ideally the biopsy should be performed before the patient is started on steroids, because the giant cells will start to shrink as soon as medication starts, and it will become increasingly likely that the biopsy won't find one, which is the 'clincher' for the diagnosis.

The GP knows that if the steroids are not started, there is a risk that the patient's sight may be damaged, or in the worst case scenario, lost altogether. There is research evidence that the presence of the giant cells can still be detected up to two weeks after the patient starts taking prednisolone, but it is a risky business. If the GP goes ahead and prescribes, there is a chance that by the time the patient sees a rheumatologist, the consultant will not be able to discern any of the signs or symptoms that would enable them to confirm or disconfirm the diagnosis. If the GP does not act and leaves the patient without the steroids, the risk is that one morning the patient will wake up unable to see. And that will be that.

The answer to this is stunningly simple, but a challenge to ensure. Patients with suspected GCA should be seen by a specialist, probably a consultant rheumatologist, immediately, ideally within 24 hours of the GP coming up with the provisional diagnosis. Increasingly, rheumatology departments are introducing fast-track systems on their own initiative. In 2012, the Department of Health gave their support to a BSR initiative to evaluate a fast-track system pioneered in the Southend area by Professor Bhaskar Dasgupta and his team. They got agreement from all the GPs in their area that any suspected cases of GCA would be reported to them immediately. In return, they provided a special emergency call service which guaranteed that any suspected case would be seen by a rheumatologist within 24 hours.

At the first international symposium on PMR and GCA, held at Chelmsford in November 2012, Dr Frances Borg outlined how the pathway works. To begin with, an audit was taken of the GCA cases referred to the local hospital since 2003. Between 2003 and 2008, there was a total of 61 patients with GCA referred to Southend University Hospital. Of these, 19, or 29% had lost vision before diagnosis. That is almost one in three. By 2010, things had hardly improved, with 26 cases in that year of which 7, or 27%, lost some or all of their sight.

The pathway plan was written by a respected local consultant, and sent out to all GPs, with the agreement of the hospital management. On suspicion of a case of GCA, the GP should make an immediate referral via a special hotline call to a GCA doctor. The GP was encouraged to start the patient on medication straight away to protect their sight. Then the patient would be seen at the GCA rapid access clinic the next working day. If it indeed looked as though the person did have GCA, they would get an appointment for both ultrasound scanning and a biopsy, which would take place within seven days. Following this, the case would be reviewed in clinic within two weeks. This means that any suspected case could be started on sight-saving medication immediately, with the assurance that the biopsy would take place within the essential two-week window for catching one of those pesky giant cells.

It worked. When the audit was done of GCA cases in 2012

up to the symposium, there had been 29 GCA cases referred to Southend University Hospital, but only one of these had suffered sight loss, and that was a person who had been referred from outside the local area. An impressive result indeed, cutting the incidence of sight loss down from 29% to 3%.

How marvellous it would be if this pattern could be repeated across the UK, and all over the world. What would be involved in making this a reality? Well, clearly, it was important for the team at Southend to secure the support of the clinical team and the hospital management. Then they had to send out the guidelines to GPs in a very simple, clear and unambiguous form. There was a certain amount of in-service training required, but the main thing was to create confidence and trust that the fast track system would actually operate as intended. It was important to be sure that the rheumatology clinic could provide the appointment within a working day, and that biopsies and ultrasound would indeed be available within the one-week 'window' specified.

The Southend process is staggeringly simple, and is just one example of fast track systems being pioneered around England and Wales. At the time of writing, an evaluation project has just reported a cost-benefit analysis of the Southend results. I tend to think that the chance to save the sight of even one person is a no-brainer. To be able to save the sight of seven or more people every year in every hospital district in the country is a total imperative. The cost-benefit analysis has reported fantastic results – not only does the fast-track system save people's sight, which in itself will save the public purse hundreds of thousands of pounds a year, but it has actually proved to be cheaper than the previous models of referral and diagnosis.

My dream is that within ten years we will be able to eradicate sight loss through late diagnosis of Giant Cell Arteritis.

Here is Sally's experience of being diagnosed with GCA, in 2012.

"During May I had begun to feel very tired, lost weight, lost my appetite. I kept being told it was a virus but as it got worse. I suspected it was something more serious.

During Jubilee weekend I began to get very painful headaches in my temples, aching jaws and face; and I noticed a swollen artery on the side of my face. My sight was a bit blurred, but I put that down to my cataracts. I rang the NHS helpline for advice on the Tuesday, and they advised me to contact out of hours to see a doctor that day. My son took me to Urgent Care, next to A and E at our local hospital.

The GP I saw did what he termed an 'MOT' on me and sounded the artery. I asked him if I had a brain tumour because I felt so ill. He said, "If you were my patient I would send you for a blood test". He made no mention of why or gave any sign of any urgency.

I made an appointment to see my own GP on June 8th. She

took tests for liver and thyroid function. Those tests were not due back until June 12th, by which time I felt so ill I had to go to the surgery and ask to be seen urgently. The GP on call recognised immediately that it was temporal arteritis (GCA), sent an urgent blood test, called me back the next day and put me on 60mg of prednisolone. He also referred me to the hospital. He told me I would go blind if I didn't take the steroids and that the GP I had seen the week before in Urgent Care had considered GCA, but because my artery pulse was normal had rejected it.

When on 29 June I attended the rheumatology clinic I asked why, if GCA was a medical emergency, had the doctor in Urgent Care not sent me for a blood test. The reply came that 'he didn't have the facility'. But Urgent Care is right next door to A and E!

Sally's story of being moved around from pillar to post is not at all unusual. I want to ask these doctors:

1. Why, when all the cardinal symptoms of GCA were present, did the GP she saw discount the suspicion of GCA based on a pulse reading?
2. Why was she not sent for a blood test?
3. Why did her own GP discount the signs and symptoms?
4. Why did the doctor who finally recognised GCA not give her 60mg of steroids immediately to safeguard her sight? She could have gone blind overnight

while waiting for the results of the blood test to come back.

5. Why did it take a further fortnight for her to be seen by a rheumatologist?

How long will I have GCA?

It probably will not surprise you to read that there are no categorical sources of information on how long people continue to have GCA. The best we can say is that the chances are that you will be on steroid therapy for two to three years. I do know of several people who have had GCA for five years or even longer. All of the points about 'remission' and 'recovery' that I made at the end of the last chapter in relation to polymyalgia rheumatica also apply to giant cell arteritis.

It is known for GCA to re-occur. I also know several people who consider themselves to be in 'remission' (although the concept of remission is problematic, as we have noted), for whom the symptoms of GCA have gone away and they are no longer on steroids or any other medication for the GCA. However, they are constantly aware and monitoring themselves for signs that it might be getting ready to stage a come-back.

Kate Gilbert

4: TREATING PMR AND GCA WITH STEROIDS

Medication Side-effects

Short-term side effects of prednisolone, as with all glucocorticoids, include fluid retention and high blood glucose levels, especially in patients with diabetes mellitus, or those on other medications that increase blood glucose. This may stabilise when the steroid dosage is reduced (but read the section on diabetes risk below).

Additional short-term side effects can include insomnia, euphoria and, rarely, mania (in particular, in those suffering from bipolar disorders). It can also cause depression or depressive symptoms and anxiety in some individuals. And yet it did not occur to me until two years after my recovery, that the awful breakdown I suffered might have been due to the steroids, because I was possibly taking more than was good for me. I do not say this lightly because I would not want to cause undue worry. If you do find that you have rather unusual mood swings early on in your treatment, do not panic. Do take some time off work to adapt to your diagnosis and your medication. If you are not working, make sure that you rest enough. Take special care of yourself and leave it a while before going back to the doctor. These unpleasant effects may wear off fairly quickly as your body gets used to the drug. Of course, if they do not wear off within a week or so, seek help from your GP.

Weight gain and 'moon face'

In the longer term, many people worry about how their appearance may change when they go on steroids. It is bad enough not feeling yourself, so not looking like yourself is like adding insult to injury. Long-term side-effects include Cushing's syndrome, which is characterised by the 'moon face' and 'buffalo hump', which are rather unflattering descriptions of the outward signs of too much corticosteroid in the body, truncal weight gain, i.e. weight gain that is confined to the trunk and not the limbs, osteoporosis, glaucoma and cataracts, type II diabetes, and possible depression on withdrawal from the steroids. The effects on the eyes (glaucoma), osteoporosis (because of the risk of falls and fractures), and diabetes are likely to be the long-term side effects that worry doctors most where elderly people are concerned. Doctors are less likely to worry about moon face and moderate weight gain, and you may get the impression that the doctor thinks you are making a fuss about it. This is one area in which getting in touch with other people, for example through a local support group, or on the web forum, can be tremendously helpful. In the company of your fellow-sufferers you can talk, rant, and laugh about your side effects, knowing that you are not alone.

Dorothy Byrne wrote an article in the Daily Mail about how difficult she found dealing with her changed appearance. As a senior creative in the media industry, she is really in a position where she is surrounded by people for whom appearance matters a lot. Dorothy shared how she found out what doctors think about the side effects of prednisolone:

"Doctors call our chubby chops 'moon face'. It's caused partly by water retention, but also by the peculiar way in which steroids redistribute fat round the body. Steroids make takers look puffier because they cause water retention and redistribute fat to the face, back and midriff

We also have little humps on our backs just below the neck, known as 'buffalo hump'. There is another weird fat deposit round our midriff. Meanwhile, our arms and legs lose muscle and fat. Some medics refer to us as 'lemons on matchsticks'. Others call us 'potatoes on sticks'. Obviously, they don't say these names to our puffy faces.

Doctors are, of course, mainly concerned with the long-term medical benefits of taking steroids and so often don't mention temporary changes in appearance to patients. I've interviewed several people who didn't know until I told them that the weird fat deposit round their torso was caused by steroids.

Similarly a lot of doctors don't, or hardly ever, mention the -

possibility that you'll put on weight. In fact, someone on long-term steroids for PMR might expect to put on half a stone.

For some patients this causes huge misery, because it is hard to get used to looking different from your 'real self' as well as feeling like hell. We get this deposit of fat in unwelcome places, like round our middles (what we used to call our 'roid rolls'), the 'buffalo hump', or 'rhino hump' (which is worse?) and the moonface, while we lose fat and muscle from our upper arms. If PMR or GCA strike during or soon after the menopause, all this change of appearance can be just too much for women who are just getting used to the idea of getting older. It is bad enough to have an illness that is supposed to be 'an illness of the elderly', without having to cope with sudden weight gain at the same time. In my own case, it did not bother me too much at the time. My husband was very sweet and reassuring, remarking on my blooming complexion instead of drawing attention to my blooming belly. But once I got better and began to look more like my old self, before PMR, I could tell by some of the things that he said that he was secretly relieved to have me back to my 'normal' self.

Increased blood sugar

Corticosteroid drugs tend to play havoc with your body's blood sugar levels. If you are a diabetic before developing PMR or GCA, you do need to be very careful indeed about monitoring your blood sugar levels and keeping them under control by taking your diabetes medication religiously.

There is also a lot you can do to help yourself and protect your overall level of health in the long term, by being even stricter about your diet. Try to restrict your refined carbohydrate (sugars) intake as much as you can. If you are relatively young when you get PMR or GCA, say in your fifties, a couple of years of relative self-denial now will pay dividends in future years by helping to keep your diabetes under control.

Even if you are not diabetic, you need to be aware of the risks. Diabetes induced by long-term corticosteroid use is a real risk. I know, because it happened to me. I was taking prednisolone for three and a half years. Six months after coming off them for good, I was feeling just as ill as I had felt with PMR, but in a different way. I had a chronic headache and was overwhelmed with a stifling fatigue. It was only when I started drinking bottled water like there was no tomorrow that it dawned on me that I might have diabetes. So when the blood test results came through, the doctor was surprised, but I was not.

Every part of our body burns energy, at different rates of course. Normally, in response to insulin, the liver decreases its output of glucose. Glucocorticoids like prednisolone decrease the liver's sensitivity to insulin, thereby inducing the liver to keep on increasing its glucose output. They also inhibit glucose uptake in muscle and fat, reducing insulin sensitivity as much as 60% in healthy volunteers. This means that the liver is churning out ever more glucose, while the pancreas is churning out insulin as hard as it can, and the glucose is going round and round in the bloodstream rather than being used up by the cells of the body. Eventually this combination of high blood glucose, strain on the pancreas and increased insulin sensitivity spills over into full-blown diabetes.

What can we do to avoid this happening? Well obviously, we need to keep our steroid intake as low as we can. We can do a lot to protect our systems by cutting down the amount of simple carbohydrate, i.e. starch, that we are eating. Starchy foods are most readily and quickly converted into glucose. So it stands to reason that in a body that has PMR and isn't well set up to burn large amounts of energy quickly, because of that combination of weight gain and relative immobility and the insulin-suppressing effects of the prednisolone, that glucose will cause dangerous spikes in the blood sugar. We will be looking more closely at this shortly in the section on nutrition in this chapter.

It is a challenge though, because often, steroids make us more hungry than we would normally be. Pass the crisps, please, would you?

Suppression of the adrenal gland

Prednisolone is chemically related to hydrocortisone, or cortisol, which in the normal healthy body is manufactured in the adrenal gland. Healthy bodies produce corticosteroids naturally, in the working of our adrenal systems. This happens during the hours of daylight and stops during the night, which is why most people take their steroid tablets first thing in the morning. Taking steroids will suppress this natural process. This mechanism leads to dependence in a short time and can be very dangerous if medications are withdrawn too quickly.

Taking prednisolone suppresses the adrenal gland so that it does not produce as much hydrocortisone as before, and may go out of production altogether. Adrenal suppression will begin to occur if prednisone is taken for longer than a week. Low levels of natural cortisol have been known to cause many symptoms, including chronic fatigue and weakness, weight loss, stomach upset, vomiting, headache and low blood pressure. This is why it is dangerous to stop taking steroids suddenly – the body will be left without a supply of cortisol, which is essential for many functions in the body.

Instead, the dosage should be gradually reduced. This weaning process may be over a few days, if the course of prednisolone was short, but may take weeks or months if the patient had been on long-term treatment.

The body must have time to begin synthesis of CRH and ACTH and for the adrenal glands to begin functioning normally again. This can take several months. It is worth considering that some of the pain and stiffness that patients report even when their blood results are normal, may be due to adrenal malfunction.

Some experts, including some in the international PMR

working group, are beginning to think that patients' age should also be taken into account regarding the adrenal system. Older patients are less able to boost their natural cortisol production. Therefore it would make sense to start their PMR treatment off at a lower dose level, which would mimic the level in a healthy person, rather than trying to 'zap' the inflammation of PMR with steroids, thus knocking out their natural cortisol production altogether.

It is worth mentioning that, as we get older, after a lifetime of our stressed-out western lifestyle, many of us may be already suffering from 'adrenal exhaustion', even without having an autoimmune illness and having to take steroids. The adrenal system has a delicate balance between cortisol, and another hormone called *Dehydroepiandrosterone* (DHEA), which helps to regulate levels of cortisol in the body. It also protects your cardiovascular system, protects against levels of 'bad' cholesterol, and protects intellectual functioning (sharpening the mind). When cortisol is up, DHEA is down. When levels of these substances get out of kilter, we experience symptoms such as sleep disturbance, cravings for sweet foods, declines in libido. Gradually, if we suffer from too much stress, our adrenal systems can become seriously exhausted. Add PMR or GCA to the mix and the need to take synthetic corticosteroids, and you have a pretty evil combination. Dr Christine Northrup, who has a website dedicated to women's health (see useful links at the end of the book), suggests that the only way to address this adrenal exhaustion is through lifestyle changes, removing the sources of chronic stress as much as possible.

When tapering down to lower doses, some doctors encourage patients to take a dose every other day, as this might have the effect of helping the adrenal glands to kick back into action (see the section on 'the sting in the tail' in Chapter 5).

Difficulty controlling emotion.

We have touched on steroid psychosis, which is unusual, but there are other emotional effects of steroids that are not uncommon. You may find you are feeling weepy, or perhaps particularly irritable, when you are taking steroids. Do talk with your nearest and dearest about the possible effects on your emotions, and tell them that at times you may exhibit mood swings. If we add to this the fact that you may be fed up because you are in pain and worn out because you have not slept very well, we have a pretty explosive mixture. Do not beat yourself up about it if you find you can't be stoical and heroic all the time. Accept yourself.

Difficulty in maintaining train of thought. This is a common one. Hmm... where was I? Many of our members in PMRGCAuk and the local support groups have complained about their 'steroid head'. As a university teacher, I found this particularly hard, and I am sure that it affected my career in the closing stages. I just did not feel that I had the intellectual sharpness I had had before PMR.

You may have difficulty making decisions. Unfortunately, as many of us are getting on, we might start to think that our lapses of memory, and drying up in the middle of a sentence having completely forgotten what we were going to say, are part of creeping decrepitude. Not so. This is the effect of the steroids. Don't give yourself a bad time about it. Just get into the habit of writing things down! Now where did I put that biro?

Effects on the eyes

Chapter 1 on PMR has mentioned eye symptoms. Many people experience changes in their eyesight while they are taking steroids, and this can be one of the most worrying side effects, particularly for people with PMR, who may wonder whether GCA is rearing its ugly head, and those with GCA, who may fear a flare-up and possible permanent damage to the eyes. However, what may be more probable is a change to the internal curvature of the eye caused by spikes in the blood sugar, due to the steroids, as we mentioned above. If you experience this, you could try cutting down your carbohydrate intake for a day or two and see whether a reduction in your blood sugar has any effect. If it happens frequently, you may need a blood test for diabetes. Another problem, especially for us older people, is glaucoma. You should have a regular ophthalmological check-up to watch out for this. Ditto cataracts.

Minor

As if all this were not enough, a whole series of side effects are characterised by medics as being 'minor'. These include nervousness, acne, rashes, increased appetite, hyperactivity, frequent urination, diarrhoea, leg cramps, and sensitive teeth. You may experience bouts of sleep disturbance while you have PMR or GCA, and it is difficult to pinpoint whether this is due to the illness itself, or the side effects of the steroids.

Tapering the steroids

Have you been having trouble getting down below 10mg per day of prednisolone? If so, you are not alone! Coming down from the initial higher doses for PMR and even for GCA may not be so difficult, but once we are down below 15mg things may start to get harder. Many of us find it incredibly hard, and discover that when we try reducing from, say, 8mg to 7mg, all our symptoms seem to come back with a vengeance. You might wonder if you are having a flare, or whether this is your body complaining about getting a lower dose. This is a stage in the journey of PMR and GCA when you may feel particularly alone. This is not what the doctor told you would happen. Up to now, you felt you were doing so well. Now, you have stopped being a 'good' patient. You ache, you can't turn over in bed, you feel wiped out. What is going wrong?

When you think about it, a drop from 8 to 7mg is just about twice as big a drop, *proportionately,* as one from 15 to 14, so it's no wonder we have trouble. The further down we go, the bigger a drop 1mg gets, as a proportion of what we were taking before.

At the first international symposium on PMR and GCA, held

in Chelmsford, Essex in 2012, a German consultant said that
he puts his patients on a very gradual reduction indeed.
This struck a chord with me and made a lot of sense, so I
want to tell you about it too.

His patients, when getting down from 8mg to 7mg daily, will
spend a week with six days on 8mg and one on 7mg. The
next week, five days on 8mg and two on 7mg (not together,
say, Sunday and Tuesday). And so on until the whole week
is on 7mg per day. This means that the reduction is a bit
slower, but the body gets fooled into not really noticing the
drop, and adapts itself to the lower dose. This is also a good
way to 'switch on' the adrenal glands that have been
dormant during steroid treatment, when the dose gets
really low, less than 5mg per day.

If you think this kind of reduction programme might suit
you, and prevent you having flares and suffering pain and
stiffness while you are reducing, why not discuss it with
your GP or consultant?

When I was struggling to reduce, and found myself 'yo-yo-
ing' up and down from 7.5mg per day, a rheumatology
nurse reminded me that painkillers are allowed. That is,
paracetamol, or for those who can take it without suffering
constipation, cocodamol. Non-steroidal anti-inflammaries
such as Ibuprofen, do not work well with PMR or GCA and
generally it is recommended that they should be avoided.
In fact, the international group working on the latest set of
guidance for PMR have decided that there should be a *very*
strong recommendation that NSAIDs are *not* used.

But as Jane said, taking the full dose of 8 x paracetamol a day (four doses of two tablets), won't hurt you, even if you take it every day for a couple of weeks. Do discuss this with your doctor, though, especially if you have, or have had, any liver or kidney problems. Obviously overdosing on paracetamol is dangerous, but for most people the recommended dose is within safe limits. I found that if I took a dose on waking up, I could sometimes make it to about 3 o'clock in the afternoon before I started to feel the pain too much again. Every time I reduced my dose from then on, I would take the paracetamol every day for about four or five days, and gave my body a chance to adapt to the lower dose.

Many of us were brought up to be stoical and to avoid painkillers as though there is something morally dubious about them. As though taking painkillers marks you out as a wimp. There is no point in this. As my doctor pointed out that time when he had to give me a particularly strong talking-to, putting up with chronic pain is the surest path to depression. Why use your psychic energy fighting pain, when you could be using it to heal yourself?

Are there any alternatives to steroids?

As part of the process of developing international guidelines for the diagnosis and management of PMR, the international working group has to gather data on patients' perceptions of the risks and benefits of medication, as compared with the symptoms of the disease. There was an interesting result when we polled members of our HealthUnlocked web forum community about their attitudes to the risk of suffering side effects. Because we tend to hear a lot about how much people hate the meds, especially steroids, and want to get off them, those of us who volunteer on the helpline and forum, and meet people at support groups, might get the idea that people think of medications as at worst the enemy, at best a necessary evil.

It was surprising to find that the overwhelming majority of voters were generally positive on balance about their medication. Out of 108 voters, three out of ten agreed strongly with the statement 'I would rather take the risks of side-effects from medication than lower my quality of life with PMR symptoms'. Another 50% of respondents were in general agreement. Around 9% of voters felt the other way – that in some ways the medication is worse than the illness.

Clearly, we have a love-hate relationship with steroids. All the more reason why, as a patient organisation, PMRGCAuk would like to see more doctors prepared to try 'steroid-sparing' drugs such as methotrexate (MTX) with PMR and GCA, to reduce the patient's overall consumption of prednisolone, as has become commonplace in the treatment of rheumatoid arthritis. Methotrexate is one of a family of drugs known as DMARDs.

Disease-modifying antirheumatic drugs (DMARDs) work to decrease pain and inflammation, to reduce or prevent joint damage, and to preserve the structure and function of the joints. DMARDs work by suppressing the body's overactive immune and/or inflammatory systems. They take effect over weeks or months and are not designed to provide immediate relief of symptoms.

The choice of DMARD depends on a number of factors, including the stage and severity of the condition, the balance between possible side effects and expected benefits, and patient preference. Before treatment begins, the patient and clinician should discuss the benefits and risks of each type of therapy, including possible side effects and toxicities, dosing schedule, monitoring frequency, and expected results.

The most common DMARDs are methotrexate, sulfasalazine, hydroxychloroquine, and leflunomide. Methotrexate (MTX) and leflunomide are the ones that have been systematically used with intransigent cases of PMR or GCA, where either steroids haven't been effective, or the patient has been unable to tolerate them.

MTX was originally used as a chemotherapy treatment for cancer. In PMR and GCA it is used in smaller doses, but many patients are still apprehensive about side effects. Common side effects include upset stomach and a sore mouth. Methotrexate can interfere with the bone marrow's production of blood cells. Low blood cell counts can cause fever, infections, swollen lymph nodes, and easy bruisability and bleeding. Liver or lung damage can occur, even with low doses, and, therefore, requires monitoring. However, clinicians say that if a patient is going to be intolerant to MTX, the side effects will appear quickly so that the medication can be quickly discontinued. This is an advantage over prednisolone in comparison, where the side effects are creeping and cumulative. People using methotrexate are strongly discouraged from drinking alcoholic beverages because of the increased risk of liver damage with this combination.

Monitoring reduces the risk of long-term damage from methotrexate. If your rheumatologist suggests MTX for you, a chest x-ray is recommended before beginning treatment, and your bloods should be taken regularly. While taking methotrexate, most patients take folic acid 1 mg daily to reduce the risk of certain side effects, such as upset stomach, sore mouth, low blood cell counts, and abnormal liver function. Some PMR and GCA patients have experienced significant improvement in their symptoms when taking MTX, and others have been able to come off steroids completely. It is likely that the new international guidelines on PMR, due to come out later in 2014, may open the way for a wider use of MTX than has been customary in the UK in the past, for 'complex' cases.

Leflunomide inhibits production of inflammatory cells to reduce inflammation. It is taken by mouth once daily. Side effects include rash, temporary hair loss, liver damage, nausea, diarrhoea, weight loss, and abdominal pain. Regular testing to monitor for liver damage is required.

Azathioprine (AZA) is another DMARD that has been used in the treatment of cancer, rheumatoid arthritis, lupus, and a variety of other inflammatory illnesses since the 1950s. It has also been used in organ transplantation to prevent rejection of the transplanted organ. AZA is generally reserved for patients who have not responded to other treatments.

It is usually taken by mouth once to four times daily. The most common side effects of AZA include nausea, vomiting, decreased appetite, liver function abnormalities, low white blood cell counts, and infection. Blood testing is recommended during treatment with AZA.

Tocilizumab is one of a new generation of 'biologic' drugs that are showing promise for the treatment of chronic inflammatory diseases. In rheumatoid arthritis, TCZ seems to suppress the body's manufacture of the cytokines such as IL-6 that cause the inflammation in the first place. And for this reason it can be thought of as treating the actual disease, rather than treating the symptoms further 'downstream'. TCZ is however very expensive indeed. It is estimated that it could cost up to £18,000 a year to treat a person with Giant Cell Arteritis, whereas the cost of treating them with steroids is almost nothing. So if the current trials of TCZ in GCA turn out to be effective, we may have a battle on our hands to get it approved for general use, or even in incalcitrant cases.

Kate Gilbert

5: LIVING WITH PMR AND GCA

Managing Pain

Different individuals have different responses to pain. In two individuals, the pain threshold and pain tolerance levels may be quite different. The pain threshold is the point at which pain starts to be felt. The level of pain tolerance is the point at which the intensity of pain becomes too much for the person experiencing it.

There is some evidence from research that men and women differ when it comes to experiencing and reporting pain. Women (in general) seem to feel pain at lower thresholds than men, and have lower tolerance levels. There are various theories about why this is the case. It may have something to do with women's emotionality, such as they may tune in to the negative feelings associated with pain more easily, or earlier, than men (in general) do. An alternative theory is that women's caring roles mean that they are biologically programmed to notice pain in themselves in case this signals an inability to care for other people. A third idea is that women's apparent increased sensitivity to pain links to levels of hormones in their bloodstreams. Whatever the 'truth' of all this, it is quite evident that being in chronic pain can sap a person's energy, leading to low mood and even clinical depression.

People tend to differ dramatically in their attitude towards taking painkillers. I have found there is a tendency in people who call the helpline, for example, to say very clearly that they do not want to take painkillers, that they would prefer to 'manage' without them. I used to be one of them but I have since changed my mind. As we noted in the last chapter, taking a couple of paracetamol a couple of times a day is not going to be as harmful as upping the steroids.

My experience with PMR was that, apart from the first couple of days on 20mg of steroids, I never had a day without pain. Pain and stiffness went hand-in-hand for me. They were the two sides of the same coin. Sometimes pain caused me more anguish, sometimes stiffness. Eventually I understood that I had to come to terms with my pain, almost make friends with it, in order to carry on.

How can you make friends with your pain? Well, I understood that it was not going to go away for a long time, and my pain and I were on a journey together. Like any travelling companion, I could pay attention to it all the time, or not. I could use mindfulness techniques to really concentrate on my pain, to 'get in touch with it'; and in doing that, I realised that, although it was very unpleasant, the pain of PMR was not going to destroy me. I am not talking here about the pain of GCA, which is a different matter altogether, by the way.

Most mornings, having paid the pain some attention, and taken a couple of paracetamol with my breakfast, I found that there were times when I could become unaware of it, although it was still there. The worst times for me were at night, when I would cry out in my sleep with pain. Had I known at that time that the levels of IL-6 were highest in my bloodstream at about two in the morning, I would have experimented with taking the paracetamol, and perhaps some of my steroids, at night.

You may find that using a TENS machine is helpful when the pain is particularly bothersome. TENS stands for 'transcutaneous electrical nerve stimulation' and works by attaching a couple of pads to the skin and stimulating the nerves by passing a small electric impulse to the affected parts of the body. I did find it worked for me to some extent, but I could never figure out whether it was actually reducing my level of pain, or whether the involuntary contractions of my muscles were just giving me some distraction!

Recently I have found meditation to be a boon. I no longer have the pain and stiffness of PMR but I still find myself getting very tense and achy, and a few minutes' relaxed meditation get me back onto an even keel. There is nothing weird or strange about meditation. For me it is technique for stilling my over-active mind and relaxing the body. I have even downloaded an app onto my smartphone that reminds me to do my meditation every day, that gives me a thought to meditate on, and times me. How good is that for a control freak!

Work

For me, one of the hardest aspects of living with PMR was coming to terms with its impact on my working life. To begin with, as a university teacher managing a large department in a business school, I did not have time to be ill. I went for weeks and weeks ignoring the worsening stiffness in my shoulders, putting it down to 'tension'. On one level, I knew I was ill, but my attention was elsewhere, until I simply could not go on any longer and my body called time on me.

At 54, I was young to get polymyalgia rheumatica, and I quickly discovered that PMR and GCA do not appear on the radar of most employing organisations. Because they are regarded as illnesses of the 'elderly' (a word PMRGCAuk is working to remove from descriptions of PMR and GCA), there has been no research on the impact that having PMR or GCA has on a person's working life. Certainly, there are worse things that can go wrong with us in middle age than getting polymyalgia rheumatica. But these illnesses are so little known and so poorly understood that people who do get them are at a real disadvantage when it comes to working out how they are going to affect them at work.

Many people think of PMR and GCA as illnesses that elderly people get. Therefore, it is easy to forget that the people who get PMR and GCA while in their 50s make up a sizeable proportion of the statistics. What is it like for people who find themselves facing these illnesses while they may be still at work, running a business, caring for children and parents, or both?

I was 54 when I first became ill with PMR. Over a period of three months I went from running at least ten miles a week, to walking with a stick, and being almost unable to haul myself out of bed. Once I was diagnosed I thought back, and realised that I had probably been feeling unwell for some time, and had had a constant headache for weeks; but I kept putting that down to the stress of my busy and high-pressured job. The steroids performed their magic and I was able to carry on working. I tried to carry on as if nothing was wrong. There was a huge physical and mental effort involved. I would have to get up in the middle of a meeting to walk around the table and stretch my crooked body out. I was not such a good listener to my colleagues and students, because the amount of physical discomfort I was in was sapping my attention. I was becoming a grumpy old woman.

After a few months, I realised that I would have to scale down, and took a job at a new place at a lower level on the career ladder. After a few months in this new job, I went part-time. This felt much better, but I had to come to terms with the fact that this was going to affect me for the rest of my life, because it would hit my income forever. Still I was one of the lucky ones – I was able to carry on working.

Since being involved with PMRGCAuk, I have heard about people like Alan, aged 55, a self-employed builder staring early retirement in the face. Anne, 56, a single parent, living in a rural area, lost her livelihood because late diagnosis of

GCA led to loss of the vision in one eye, and she could no longer drive to the college where she taught.

Julie, aged only 52, has found that she cannot manage a part-time job and family, and have a social life as well. Something has to give. Julie has had to explain to friends that she cannot join them for evenings in the pub. "I can manage to go out about once a week. I can even manage a pub meal, but before getting ill I could dance till one o clock in the morning, and keep up with the best of them. I did manage a couple of dances the other week, but I was completely good for nothing the next day. And I have my two teenage sons to cook and keep house for."

Although she was of an 'average' age when she got PMR, at74, June, of Southend, was far from average. She was still working full-time in the family restaurant business, and felt that she could not give up working. "One just had to put it to one side and get on with it", she says. "If you give in to it you just get worse." June is convinced that working actually helped her through the PMR because it kept her more supple than she would have been if she had been retired and at home. "I had bad days, but fortunately it went." June admits she was determined – "determined to get rid of it!" Her advice to people who get PMR while they are working is not to give up work. PMR can make you miserable, she says, and if you give up work this can make it worse. June, like many others, has been left with shoulder pain after PMR, but she feels better now, and at 80 has finally retired.

Wendy, who is a PMRGCAuk Trustee, says that she has only been able to keep going because she works just three days a week in a desk job. This was as much as she could manage, especially bearing in mind that she combines her job with family life and a demanding volunteer schedule. 'I arranged the office so that nothing was handy', she says. "I had to get up from the desk to get anything, so that I wouldn't sit still for too long, which is so easy to do when you are absorbed in what you are doing." In the early days Wendy would experience a sudden lethargy "like hitting a brick wall", and would find that her head did not wake up till late in the morning, and would not want to work after about four in the afternoon. "So I planned all meetings to be between 11 and 4 and would only do routine work at the start and end of every day."

So getting PMR or GCA while you are still of working age is no joke. It has a massive effect on all aspects of your life. Having listened to lots of people now, I would say to anybody 'Don't try to pretend that nothing has happened and carry on regardless. If you have help at hand, like an Occupational Health department, use it. A good employer may even be pleased to know about your illness because, as far as they are concerned, if they can help you it shows that they are fulfilling the requirements of the Disability Discrimination Act. I was amazed to find that I became a 'good' statistic as far as my employer was concerned. It was a relief to 'come out' and admit that I needed help to be able to carry on doing my job.

As people work longer and longer, there will be more and

more people bringing PMR and GCA to work. However, we have a long way to go before employers really understand the help and support people need when they get PMR or GCA during their working lives.

Do you find that you cannot keep the house as clean and tidy as it used to be? We all know that keeping the house nice is not the most important thing in the world. However, it certainly helps, when you are feeling down, to be in a pleasant environment. Many people with PMR say that things are getting on top of them. We asked other people with PMR and GCA for their tips on keeping on top of housework rather than letting it get on top of you. Here are their ideas!

a) Keep a small basket at the bottom of the stairs. When you think of something you need to take upstairs pop it in the basket until you need to go up anyway.

b) Get rid of heavy pottery storage jars (even if they are pretty) and replace them with lightweight plastic ones.

c) Have a good clearout. Cut down the amount of clutter in your home that is attracting dust. A good clearout can be fantastically uplifting. If you feel that some things have memories for you, take a photo of that thing – the memories will still be there. Make sure you have some help to get unwanted things out of the house. Give it to charity.

d) Keep a packet or two of surface wipes handy around the house. They really are good at picking up dust and sticky marks. Much less trouble than lugging a bowl of water around.

e) If you have room, keep a second lightweight vacuum cleaner upstairs.

f) Wipe down the tiles in the shower after you have showered. Clean the bathroom in the nude and then treat yourself to a lovely long soak.

g) Do one room completely, one at a time. Don't try to do more than one room a day. Then, if one room is a mess, you can go into the room that you have done and give yourself a big pat on the back (well, metaphorically anyway)

h) Do you have a space upstairs near the bathroom? Plumb the washing machine in upstairs and move the drier up too if you have one. Take the ironing board and iron upstairs too. Use a spare bedroom as a utility room. Saves lots of trudging up and down stairs with piles of dirty and clean washing. And it keeps it all out of sight.

i) Cut down the amount of bedding you have to wash. Use a top sheet under the duvet cover. This saves washing the duvet cover too often. When you change the sheets, this top sheet becomes the bottom sheet. This way, you only have to wash one sheet at a time. Don't even think about ironing them!

j)   If you have an adult son or daughter, jot down a note of things they can do for you next time the come to see you. Don't feel guilty about asking. They are usually happy to do something for you, it gives them a warm glow.

k)   Don't be afraid to ask for help from family and friends. They need to understand that you are unwell, even if they think you look marvellous, with your disappearing wrinkles and blooming skin.

Let's get physical

This section has been one of the most difficult to think about, before writing. We are all different, and making generalisations about what physical activity people could or should do could be foolish, and even dangerous. Clearly, the issues involved in physical activity and maintaining physical mobility are different if one is 83 or 53 at diagnosis. Then, we all have different starting points. I know many 70-year-olds who are fitter and more energetic than several 40-year-olds of my acquaintance.

Before I became ill with PMR, I was a runner. I had run the London Marathon at the age of 49, and had carried on doing occasional half-marathons. So at 54, I was pretty fit. However, PMR put paid to that, and I had to scale down to walking. I could still go on a long walk of about six miles, but I could only do it once a week. I could still manage a swim, but only half as many lengths as I could do before. And after each day that I exercised, I would need to have a rest day.

John Robson of Durham is a phenomenon. A senior fire service officer, he is well known both locally and nationally for his magnificent fund-raising accomplishments, through taking on extreme physical challenges like marathon running and climbing. John's idea of a perfect holiday is climbing five peaks in Kazakhstan in one go, and before falling ill with PMR at the age of 51, he was preoccupied with shaving a few minutes off his time every time he did another marathon. Now, John is a year and a half into his treatment for PMR, and has started running again. For runners, feeling the ground moving under your feet is one of the most wonderful and even spiritual experiences possible, something that we long for even when we are unable to do it. I have discussed this will to run with John, and he and I seem to be in agreement with this principle. While you are healthy, you can try to push your body just beyond its limits. When you are recovering from polymyalgia (and perhaps GCA as well), you can only work your body within its limits. But gradually those limits will expand. John is keeping a detailed log of his physical activities so that he can track his progress, however small the steps in that progress may be.

I think I hear some readers uttering a hollow laugh at the prospect of going out for a run. I am not trying to suggest hat we should all be rushing off to get fit as an athlete. Far from it. Rather, that whatever our level of physical activity was before we got ill and before we went onto medication, we could think in terms of maintaining that activity, but at a fraction, maybe half, of the level we did it at before. Then make sure that we build in sufficient recovery time afterwards.

The body has 205 bones and 650 muscles. When you think of it this way, it is a wonder that we don't have more things go wrong with us than we already do! Billy Fashanu, Consultant Physiotherapist at Southend University Hospital, gave some invaluable tips on how to take better care of ourselves when PMR brings us low with its horrible chronic pain.

To begin with, we can learn to use physical activity to help us manage the pain, once we have got ourselves sorted out with medication. Different forms of exercise have different functions, and Billy told us that we should think of exercise in the following order: Stretch, Move, Strengthen (Power), Balance and Rest. Although rest comes last in this sequence, it certainly does not come least, and for that reason, I am going to talk about it first.

Rest

For the body to repair itself and recover, rest is essential after exercise and other forms of physical activity. There is not a great deal of point in starting an exercise regime if you are not getting enough rest. Which means getting a good night's sleep, and taking a nap during the day if necessary. My mum, who is now in her 80s, takes a nap religiously for half an hour every afternoon. The other day she reminded me that this habit started when *she* had PMR, over 25 years ago. I was at work and was unable to take a nap. Maybe that goes some way to explaining how Mother managed to recover in two years, while it took me four and a half.

Posture when lying down is also important. If we lie on our side, our legs and spine get out of alignment. The weight of the leg on top pushes downwards, compressing the lower part of the body. This distortion then carries through to the rest of our bodies, so we are constantly shifting around trying to find a more comfortable position. Billy suggests sleeping with a pillow between our knees to keep the legs and the hips aligned.

For back sleepers, the problem can be due to arching of the lower back. Again, the trusty pillow comes into service, this time underneath the knees. This can make an amazing difference to back and neck comfort in bed.

No amount of pillow talk will make any difference if the mattress has had it. Billy's advice is that a mattress, even a good one, only has a life of about 10 years. So if you are sleeping on an old mattress and have PMR, get yourself sorted out with a new one! It may be quite an investment to have to make, but it could pay dividends in a quicker and more complete recovery. Not to mention the other health benefits of having a good night's sleep. It does not need to be a hard orthopaedic mattress. The most important thing is that it should give support to the whole body, all of the time. Many older people prefer a slightly softer mattress and this can be better because it allows the body to sink in where it needs to.

Stretch

After a good rest, we need a good stretch to get us going again. Most animals stretch. It is part of keeping the body well, and it feels good. Billy and other physios recommend having a good stretch every day as a kind of systems check. It works by regaining and maintaining adequate flexibility. If you cannot move, you lose your mobility. Simple. The degree of mobility that you have determines the quality of your life. Billy goes further. Mobility is life itself. We cannot survive without it.

Lying on your back, flex your knees one at a time, drawing them up towards your chest. Use your arms to pull your leg towards your torso. Next, try stretching each leg up towards the ceiling, bringing them down slowly with knee bent.

For hips, spine and shoulders, try this sequence: get onto all fours like a cat. Take your time about getting down there! When you feel stable, keeping your back as horizontal as you can, push your backside backwards, keeping your hands still and letting your arms stretch. Start to drop your rear end down near your feet, let your head fall down between your arms, and feel that good stretch all through your body.

Come back up slowly and gently.

You should feel an immediate sense of well-being as your blood starts flowing better round your body, and you are giving your joints and muscles a good tune-up.

Move

When it comes to exercise, Billy talks about an exercise 'road map' for patients. Clearly, there is no point in advising an elderly person with mobility problems to go and have a game of squash. The first step is simply to reduce sedentary activities. Less sitting around, in other words, and more moving about, even if it is only moving around the house. Then, gradually, increase your level of *moderate* activity. Take your time over this, but the objective is to achieve periods of brisk walking with noticeable increases in pulse and breathing rate. Getting a bit out of breath is good. Billy's view is that there can and should be less emphasis on the ideal of attaining high levels of activity. The idea of having to do 30 minutes of intense activity five times a week is not only unrealistic, but unnecessary. He is at pains to emphasise that everyday activities like going up to the loo, or putting the cat out, do not count as 'moderate physical activity'.

'Good' forms of exercise include stepping up and down, walking, exercising in a pool, if this is comfortable, and riding a cycle machine.

Strengthen

As you get used to moving more, you will gradually start to get stronger. Of itself, PMR does not weaken your muscles, but the combination of immobility and steroids will have that effect. You do not need to pump iron in the gym. Just try simple weight training with a couple of tins of beans to start with. Start with side curls.

Take a tin of beans or soup in each hand, arms relaxed to your sides. Gently pull your forearms up in an arc to your shoulders, keeping your upper arms close in to your body. Hold it for a couple of seconds and release. Repeat ten times. If you do this twice a day every day, you will soon start to feel and see some improvement. Who knows, you may soon be waving those bingo wings goodbye!

Balance

Balance in later life becomes incredibly essential, as we all want to avoid falls. Try this heel raise exercise for starters. Stand tall holding a sturdy chair, table or the sink. Raise your heels taking your weight over your big toe. Hold for a second. Lower your heels with control. Repeat 10 times.

Some people find that going to see a physiotherapist is one of the best things they can do when recovering from PMR and GCA. A good physiotherapist can help your mobility by carrying out a careful assessment. He or she can also advise you on the right exercises and moves to maintain your flexibility and keep your muscle strength. Sometimes long-term steroid use can lead to damage to the 'soft tissues' such as the ligaments and tendons. People occasionally find that, when their PMR is getting better, they experience a different kind of pain in one or both shoulders. This is a sharp pain when moving the shoulder, particularly when raising the arms (rotator cuff problems). A physiotherapist can help prevent or treat these problems.

Nutrition

As PMR and GCA are inflammatory conditions, many people ask whether there are any dietary changes they can make to reduce inflammation in the body. Take this information as a guide only, as there is no established research evidence regarding treatment of PMR and GCA with diets or supplements. I can say this with some confidence, because the international group working on the PMR guidelines have carried out an exhaustive literature search and have not been able to find any reputable reliable research on the topic.

This is not to say that there is no 'common sense' or common wisdom about the role of nutrition in health and recovery from illness. The most common way to treat PMR and GCA is taking steroids. During the acute stage, the medication is indispensable. However, after the acute stage, some people opt for helping themselves towards recovery through diet and exercise, in the hope that this will enable them to reduce their steroid intake or eliminate it altogether. Before you plan to do so, I strongly advise that you review all diet-related issues with your GP or rheumatologist.

In the information available on PMR and GCA, such as the ARUK leaflets, there is quite a lot of emphasis placed on the risk of developing osteoporosis when you are on steroids. This is a real risk, and you should take a calcium supplement and be sure to eat foods that are rich in calcium. The Mayo Clinic, for instance, recommends incorporating whole grains, sufficient calcium and vitamin D, as well as low-fat meat. This could help to prevent potential problems such as thinning bones, high blood pressure and diabetes. Several rheumatologists also recommend oily fish such us sardines, herring, trout and wild salmon. All this adds up to a low inflammatory diet.

According to the British Dietetic Association, an ideal calcium intake for adults is between 700mg and 1000mg daily. To assess how much calcium you are taking in, use the table below. Each 'point' equates to 50mg of calcium, so you should be aiming for at least 14 points a day:

Points	Calcium sources
5	1 pot plain or fruit yoghurt Or one third pint milk or 2 oz (half a tin) of sardines in tomato sauce, or 50g (2 oz) tofu.
4	1oz (30g) Cheddar cheese, or 1 oz (30g) Edam cheese, or a large serving of dark leafy green veg e.g spinach, or one third pint soya milk (calcium enriched)

3	1tblsp grated Parmesan cheese, or 2 oz tinned pilchards in tomato sauce, or 1 scoop dairy icecream, or 3 dried figs, or2 slices white or wholemeal bread, or a small pot of calcium-enriched soya yoghurt.
2	1 pot fromage frais, or half a small tin of salmon, or 4 oz (small tub) cottage cheese, or small bar milk chocolate, or half a large tin kidney beans.
1	One-third pint soya milk or 3 heaped tsp Horlicks, or 1 small tin baked beans, or 9 Brazil nuts, or 8 dried apricot halves, or 5oz boiled cabbage.

Adequate vitamin D is also important to maintain bone strength. We need vitamin D to enable us to extract the calcium from our food. Unfortunately, almost everyone in the UK is vitamin D deficient to some degree or another. The housebound are particularly vulnerable because their bodies are not making vitamin D in response to sunlight. Even use of sunscreen over factor 8 can reduce vitamin D production by as much as 80%. Dietary sources of vitamin D include oily fish, liver, egg yolks, fortified juices and some breakfast cereals, and vitamin-D enriched milk. If you are on steroids you should also be taking a vitamin D supplement, but even when you come off the steroids, continue keeping the supplement up, especially if you are over the age of 70 or have dark skin.

There is another risk, which is as serious as osteoporosis,

and that is Type 2 diabetes. Many people worry about weight gain when they are on steroids. However, it is just as important, or even more important, to lower carbohydrate intake in order to prevent rapid swings in your blood sugar level. Prednisolone is a glucocorticosteroid, and that means that it raises the glucose level in your blood, potentially placing a strain on your system and increasing the risk of diabetes.

Although I have never carried a great deal of weight, and just put on a stone while I was on steroid therapy for PMR, I ended up being diagnosed with Type 2 diabetes a few months after finishing on steroids. This was a major shock, and I felt quite resentful that nobody had warned me this might happen. I was only 58 and intending to live at least another 30 years, so the prospect of having to take diabetes medication for the rest of my life did not appeal.

As soon as you are put on steroids you should try to restrict your intake of refined sugars, i.e. cakes, biscuits and confectionery; and starchy foods, such as potatoes, rice and bread. This can be difficult when the steroids are making you hungry, so fill up instead on good quality protein foods and fruit and vegetables that don't have high carbohydrate content. We do need carbohydrates to provide the fuel that our body runs on, so it is not a good idea to try to cut them out altogether. However, some carbs are absorbed very quickly into the bloodstream, and cause 'spikes' in our blood sugar levels, putting a strain on our systems, and other carbs are absorbed more slowly. New potatoes have 'better' carbs than old potatoes, and wholemeal bread is better than processed white bread. Adjusting your carbohydrate intake will not necessarily help you recover from PMR or GCA, but will help to make sure that you are in good shape when you do recover.

Do not think that because you are getting older, and not growing or reproducing any more, you don't need protein. All of us need a certain amount of protein to help repair damaged cells and maintain optimum working of the various systems in our bodies. Some nutritionists suggest that red meats can increase inflammation in the body, and advocate getting your protein from organic, free-range chicken and fish from sustainable sources.

We have all become very used to the litany from health professionals that we need to increase our intake of fresh fruits and vegetables – the famous 'five a day'. It does seem that for us, whole fruits and veg are better than a concentrated glass of juice. This is because a glass of, say, orange juice, contains the sugars of the fruit in concentration, and fruit sugar, or fructose, is absorbed very quickly by the body. Better to eat the orange segments, because of the fibre that is included. When it comes to vegetables, just about any vegetables are really good for us, and the best thing we can do is ensure a good balance between roots, such as swedes, turnips and carrots; leaves, such as cabbage and chard; stems such as celery and asparagus; seeds, such as peas and beans; and fruits, such as tomatoes and peppers.

Vegetables are of course bursting with vitamins and

minerals, as well as fibre. Keep fresh vegetables in the fridge to improve keeping prevent loss of nutrients. It has become common knowledge that some of the vitamin content of vegetables is lost in the cooking water. Vitamin C, being water-soluble, is the most vulnerable of the vitamins from this point of view. Others, such as the fat-soluble Vitamins E and K, are not so likely to be lost. When boiling vegetables, use as little water as you can get away with. Try steaming or microwaving them instead. Microwaving works by polarizing water molecules in the food, and because the cooking times are shorter, any increased heat damage is balanced out by the quicker cooking. Contrary to popular opinion, cooking vegetables thoroughly won't necessarily reduce their nutritional value *when you eat them*. You might reduce the nutritional content to some extent, but when a vegetable is properly cooked, your digestive system will be more able to extract all the goodness from it. So if you have a delicate digestion and prefer your vegetables cooked rather than raw, do not worry about it.

Many people experiment with certain foods and substances that are claimed to reduce inflammation in the body. For example, curcumin, which is a substance in the spice turmeric, has been observed in experimental conditions to have an effect on the C-reactive protein that is a sign of inflammation in the body. However, nobody really knows how much curcumin you should eat in a 'normal diet' to make a difference, or quite what the mechanism is that is reducing the CRP.

Other foods, such as members of the solanum, or nightshade, family, are thought by some people to make inflammation worse. These foods are peppers (capsicums), aubergines, tomatoes and potatoes. Unfortunately, these last two are important ingredients in the diet of many older British people! I have done some research into this and, to be honest, I have not been able to find a single published peer-reviewed paper supporting the idea that these vegetables increase inflammation in the body. Certain websites claim that this scientific research exists while not telling us what it is. I followed one link on such a website back to another site that presented a published paper – from 1993. This reported secondhand about inflammation observed in livestock after they had been eating the stems and leaves of plants from the solanum family. However, we are not livestock. Thankfully, our diets are a bit more varied than the diet of the average cow. What is more, the concentration of the alkaloid substance that is the source of this concern is much lower in the fruits and roots of these plants than in the stems and leaves. This is because the substance is part of the plant's defence system, giving leaves and stems a bitter taste to repel the bugs. I am not about to start eating tomato leaves, so I'm not going to worry about this, and I will carry on enjoying tomatoes and even the odd aubergine. These foods are full of nutritious value, including anti-oxidants that protect bone health and other aspects of our body's amazing systems.

This is not to say, of course, that there aren't certain people who have an inbuilt sensitivity to certain foods, foods that literally 'disagree' with them. So if you can afford it, it might be worth your while trying to find out which foods might make you feel worse, and which might make you feel better. The way to do this is to cut out certain food groups (dairy, nightshades, wheat, for example) from your diet for three to four weeks. This will give your system time to eliminate any traces of those food groups and find a new 'equilibrium'. Keep a diary of your symptoms during this time. Then introduce the foods again, one at a time, for one day at a time. Then monitor for two days. So, for example, you might introduce bread on Tuesday, and monitor yourself on Wednesday and Thursday for reactions. Then on Friday, try a different food. This way of identifying what you may be intolerant to is exhaustive, and you need to plan and be very organized and *stick to it.* It might be fun, and it could give you really valuable information about your personal dietary 'do's and don'ts'. Detailed information on how to do the elimination diet experiment is available on http://www.precisionnutrition.com/elimination-diet.

At PMRGCAuk we are not able to endorse any approach in particular to managing your diet. We are a health charity and so we have to be led by the evidence, and unfortunately, the evidence on dietary changes just isn't broad enough or rigorous enough for us to recommend you to spend your money on any special foods or supplements. However, when you have PMR or GCA you can feel powerless and at the mercy of the illness and the steroids. It is important to take control and feel that you are doing whatever you can to help yourself towards recovery. I know several people who are certain that following an 'anti-inflammatory' diet is helping them. Making sensible changes to make sure that you are eating a good well-balanced diet is one of the most empowering things you can do. Just don't take it too seriously, and give yourself the occasional treat. You deserve it!

And finally, on a personal note, allow me to share with you what I believe about eating when you have a chronic health condition. I am no nutritional expert but I have read a lot, listened a lot, and thought a lot about it. And eaten a lot too! It basically boils down to a few principles:

1. Make sure you eat enough. Eat at least three times a day, preferably four, including a little snack before bedtime to help you through the night.

2. Keep your food varied. A little bit of everything and everything in moderation.

3. When you go out for a restaurant meal, go for the starter and the main, but pass on the dessert. Restaurants make big profits on puddings that are full of fat and sugar, bought in, and frankly, not very nice. Be kind to yourself and give them a miss. After a while, you won't miss them and if you do have a portion of pavlova, it will make you feel nauseous.

4. When facing something that's very fatty, however delicious it looks, picture in your mind the fat in that dish as a lump of lard sitting in the middle of your plate. Will you eat it? No of course you won't!

5. No diets while you have a chronic illness. No fasting, no 5:2 diet, no anything. Just good simple food and enough of it. Crash dieting will put your body under stress and that will just upset your immune system even more.

6: UNDERSTANDING AUTOIMMUNE ILLNESSES

The idea of 'autogens'

Newly diagnosed patients are often looking for a 'cause' of their illness, perhaps something in the environment that has triggered it. The evidence that PMR and GCA is linked to environmental factors is not available, although there are arguments put forward that autoimmune illnesses in general might be linked to environmental factors. If PMR and GCA were linked to environment, we might expect to see it affecting a wider age group, and also possibly affecting people in differently in different socio-economic groups. But a recent study by the Keele University primary care research group found no link between PMR and socio-economic status. Let us have a look though at the arguments for an environmental factor.

In her book *The Autoimmune Epidemic* Donna Jackson Nakazawa describes these chronic autoimmune conditions as 'an escalating medical crisis'. It does seem to be the case that these illnesses really got going in the last century, and were little known before the age of mass industrialization.

Could there be a link between autoimmune illnesses and the way we live today? Nakazawa points to the rise in the prevalence of MS in European countries at the rate of 3% a year since the 1960s. It is of course unclear why these higher rates are being reported. It might be to some extent because doctors are more aware of these illnesses and therefore more likely to spot them. Nakazawa is convinced that it is also due to the massive increase in the use of industrial chemicals in all manufacturing processes since the end of the second world war. These chemicals include pesticides, detergents, coatings such as Teflon for everything from saucepans to raincoats, and flame-retardent chemicals that are impregnating fabrics and fibres in almost everything we buy, from cosmetics to carpets. Nakazawa doesn't pull her punches:

"For nearly half a century, as big industry flourished, scientists sat idle in the lull of a gathering storm, not only missing today's autoimmune disease epidemic in the making but blinded to its possible causes."

She has coined the term *'autogen'* to describe a substance that might trigger an autoimmune imbalance in the body in the same way that a *carcinogen* might trigger cancer cells to grow. Silica is an example of an autogen because in certain individuals it might induce scleroderma. Autogens might include insecticides, dioxin, mercury, cadmium and benzene, to name a few. These toxic chemicals find their way into our bodies via food, our skin, and the air we breathe. As they are not part of the 'natural' environment that the human body evolved to survive in, the body is unable to rid itself of the toxic load, which accumulates over time. Eventually critical mass is reached, and the body becomes ill, in any one of a hundred possible ways.

Is it in the genes?

Genetic factors are involved in autoimmune disease. Dr Noel Rose, Chairman of the American Autoimmune Related Diseases Association, suggests that our genetic makeup accounts for about 50% of our risk of developing an autoimmune condition. It is well known that white people are more likely to develop PMR than black people. Dr Richard Watts has demonstrated that PMR is more common in the east of England than the west, which might also indicate a genetic influence. However, it is not as simple as identifying the single gene responsible. We cannot point the finger and say 'Ah…. It's *that* gene that has caused me to have PMR'. Rather a cluster of genes are *collectively* responsible for determining our *susceptibility* to autoimmunity. The level of knowledge among scientists is not yet at the stage of being able to predict who is likely to get what autoimmune condition. It is still a lottery, but what is clear is that a predisposition to autoimmune conditions runs in families. If you are diagnosed with an autoimmune illness, at some point the doctor has probably asked you whether anybody else in your family has one. The autoimmune lottery also depends not only on genetics but the other 50% of the risk is down to what we are exposed to in the way of environmental factors.

"Leaky gut syndrome"

Another theory about the reason why our immune systems go into overdrive is the possibility of a phenomenon known as 'leaky gut syndrome'. Our intestines, as we will remember from our human biology lessons at school, are in two parts. There is the small intestine, which absorbs nutrients from food, and the large intestine that processes the leftovers into waste and expels the waste from the body. The 'leaky gut' idea concerns the small intestine. Obviously, the lining of the gut needs to be permeable to allow nutrients to enter the bloodstream, but not so permeable that anything else can get in. The essence of the theory is that, in some people, perhaps due to illness, or toxins getting into the body, perhaps just due to wear and tear, tiny perforations develop in the wall of the gut that are large enough to allow microscopic particles of food into the bloodstream. As soon as these start to circulate around the body, antibodies start to go on red alert. There are foreign bodies in the bloodstream! This creates a reaction, and hey presto! – inflammation. The chronic nature of the problem means that the immune system is in a constant state of high alert.

Not surprisingly, the proponents of this theory also have a 'cure'. The suggestion is that, if we can give our small intestines a chance to heal, so that the perforations disappear and the foreign particles stop circulating, our immune systems will get the message that they don't need to be on red alert any longer and can calm down. The result will be reduced inflammation and reduced susceptibility to autoimmune conditions of all sorts. And the remedy could be pure aloe juice.

Pure aloe juice.

All kinds of claims are made for the wonderful therapeutic properties of the aloe plant, and it certainly does seem to be a potent aid to healing, say of wounds and burns. Could it also have the same effect on the inside of the body? Some people are convinced that it does, when used in its purest form, the gel-like juice from the leaves.

Aloe in this pure form is quite expensive. At time of writing (2014) a one-litre bottle costs about £21, and taking 2 fluid ounces daily will mean that the bottle lasts for about a month. The idea is that one should take the daily dose for about four months to give the digestive system time to heal. So we are talking here of an investment of about £80, or US$120, to find out whether or not it could do you any good at all.

Do not expect your doctor to support you in trying any kind of experiment with aloe juice. The most you can expect from your doctor is the observation that there might be a placebo effect. Which in any case is better than nothing, isn't it? The medical profession works on published research evidence, rather than hearsay or anecdotal evidence, and the evidence for 'leaky gut syndrome' just is not there, at least at the level that would convince scientists. It is an attractive theory because it has a kind of *face validity,* i.e. it sort of makes sense, and the lay person can understand the idea. I personally find it quite plausible.

Might it not be the explanation we have all been looking for? However, the studies that would prove the validity of the theory haven't been done, so it remains an untested, and possibly untestable, hypothesis.

If you think that the investment is worth a try, then by all means have a go at taking two fluid ounces of pure aloe juice every day and see at the end of four months whether you feel any better. To make this make any sense at all, you would need to establish a 'baseline' by taking some 'objective' measures of how you were at the start of the experiment in terms of:

- Your ESR and CRP rates
- Your daily dose of steroids
- Your level of morning stiffness, on a scale of 1 to 5
- A measure of how long your morning stiffness lasts before wearing off
- How physically restricted you are
- How many times you wake up in the night because of pain or discomfort
- Any other measures you feel are relevant to you.

At this point, I feel I should own up. I did the aloe juice experiment myself. This was when I was reducing from 5mg prednisolone per day and trying desperately to come off the pred, having been on it for three years. I had been stuck on this dose for months and could not seem to reduce it. I was miserable because I was still in considerable pain. I was still effectively disabled, in that there were still certain everyday things that I was unable to do. One thing that used to bug me was not being able to reach to the back of the kitchen cupboards under the worktop. It would take me ages to get down onto my hands and knees, and then to get up again, I would crawl to a kitchen chair to haul myself up.

Now, I am not claiming any miracles, but after the four months, I was down to 1mg prednisolone per day. One day I actually stood up off the kitchen floor by myself *without even thinking about it.* Many people have asked me, 'Do you think it was the aloe juice that helped you?' The only thing I can say in response is 'I really don't know. It might have, but I do not know how I would have been if I had not taken it.' Let us face it; the odds are that I was probably getting better anyway. The juice may have had a placebo effect. There might have been a different psychological effect – I was taking control of my condition and doing something structured to help myself. Not surprising if I felt better. It sure did not do me any harm. And I don't begrudge a penny that I spent on it.

What can we do?

Because the charity works under the advice of a Medical Advisory Panel, and we are supporters of an evidence-based approach to PMR and GCA, the policy of PMRGCAuk is not actively to endorse or promote any particular food supplement or substance that is not supported by an established body of scientific or clinical evidence. Just as one swallow does not make a summer, one research article does not make a cure, or even a treatment. We suffer from lack of evidence on three counts. Firstly, little is known generally about autoimmune illnesses, and there is no specialism of autoimmunology'. Secondly, PMR and GCA are notoriously under-researched compared with, say, rheumatoid arthritis. And thirdly, there is insufficient reliable scientific research on the positive or negative effects of food items on the symptoms of the body, other than the Big Three, fat, sugar and salt. We have to be sceptical about the potential for nutritionists to be biased.

The classical western scientific approach is to test a hypothesis, not to prove that a theory is correct, but to try to disprove it. It is only when scientists have tested a theory many times and failed to disprove it that the 'truth' of the theory can be firmly established. Anybody who has a vested interest in 'proving' something to be true, like the purveyors of food supplements for example, needs to be treated with some scepticism.

In the face of the possible onslaught of autogen pollution in our daily environment, Donna Jackson Nakazawa devotes just three pages in her long book to suggestions for what we can do to protect ourselves and give our immune systems a boost. Suggesting that trying to avoid all autoimmune triggers would be just overwhelming, she counsels concentrating on four main areas of behaviour that might give the biggest advantage with the least disadvantages to living a normal life.

The first is to *clean green.* Modern cleaning products are powerful because they contain powerful chemicals. The US

Environmental Protection Agency has suggested that the air in some homes in America might be five times more polluted than the air outside, simply because of the overuse of chemical cleaners. Using eco-friendly cleaners may be one way to protect our health as well as the planet. Alternatively, you could experiment with 'natural' cleaners such as vinegar and lemon juice. And good old water.

Secondly, think hard and read the label before you slap stuff on your skin. Another American study of 15000 cosmetic products found that almost 80% contained substances known to be harmful. Even so-called 'natural' products might be found to contain a lot of 'unnatural' ingredients along with the cucumber juice or royal jelly that gives it the 'natural' label. The main culprits in cosmetic ingredients are substances used as preservatives. When you think about it, isn't it rather amazing that a jar of face cream can go on for months without the contents turning rather yellow and unpleasant? Many perfumes and colognes also contain strong chemicals such as phthalates and parabens. Nail polishes contain phthalates, parabens, and toluene, a solvent to keep the polish flowing. If you can bear it, stop wearing perfumes. Stop dyeing your hair. Nakazawa claims that women who use dark hair dye have three times the risk of developing lupus compared with women who do not. As well as protecting ourselves, perhaps we should also be educating our daughters and granddaughters to be more careful about what they paint, rub and spray onto their bodies.

The third area where we can do something to help

ourselves is to protect ourselves from infection from surfaces and objects that we touch. Nakazawa suggests that we do not wash our hands often enough, or for long enough. Twenty seconds is the time it takes to get our hands clean, according to the US Center for Disease Control. Wash your hands often, particularly if you have a cold and are using tissues or a handkerchief. Always wash hands before eating. Do not use pens lying around in the doctor's surgery or the bank if you ever need to sign anything – carry a pen around with you and only use that. These precautions will just ease the load on your already over-taxed immune system.

Finally, get into the habit of making informed choices about how you behave as a consumer. Go to organic dry-cleaners (if you can find one), buy fresh organic food whenever you can, and ideally, food produced near to where you live. Think about the consumer choices you make and whether they will increase or potentially reduce your exposure to harmful chemicals.   The trick here is to do all this in a way that makes us feel optimistic about the world we live in rather than fearful and pessimistic. Feeling afraid is not good for our poor immune systems either. We all need to find the right balance in our lives, and nobody can tell us how to do that but ourselves.

7: RESTORING YOUR HEALTH

Keeping a positive outlook

It can be very difficult to keep a positive outlook when you have PMR or GCA. You have been experiencing pain, fear and anxiety, and often a sense of isolation. Because of our age group, having PMR and GCA can also go along with some of the difficult adjustments we have to make as we grow older. Our relationships may have changed or are changing. Our bodies are changing; we are beginning to look old. Many of us have suffered immense loss and hardship before falling ill. I have been surprised at how many women, on phoning the helpline, have told us that they were widowed perhaps a year or six months before falling prey to PMR or GCA. Others, men and women, are under stress from the responsibility of being a carer, perhaps for a spouse or an aged parent.

PMR and GCA are not just 'the aches and pains of getting older'. Your body is trying to tell you that it has all got too much. So how can you keep a positive outlook in these circumstances?

Jean Miller, who set up the Tayside support group that

became PMR-GCA Scotland, put it very succinctly when she said, "It helps if you can accept what you can do each day, even if it's only breathing. One of the hardest lessons I had to learn was that a job does not have to be finished in one go, or even two goes. It used to take me three days to do one hour's ironing. Remember that the condition does get better." (Quoted in *Arthritis,* by Gill Carrick, p.52)

We are all different, and I don't claim in this chapter to have any one-size fits all answers. Having spoken now with many people, and listened to and read their stories, I feel that it the starting point is to forgive ourselves for falling ill. Stop asking yourself why it happened. Nobody knows why it happened. It could have been almost anything that initially through your immune system into overdrive – an infection, a bereavement, an overload of stress at work, a difficult relationship. Just decide for yourself what it might have been. Look it straight in the face, acknowledge that you could not have done anything to prevent it; and move on. Let it go. Do not beat yourself up about it. Do not berate yourself for having to take medication. You will not get better without the medication. Do not blame every symptom you ever have on your PMR or GCA, or on the steroids, for that matter. You are still a normal human being, prey to viruses, bugs and any of the other hazards that life throws in our way. You are not defined by your PMR or GCA and it does not own you.

Tell yourself every day that *you will get better* – regaining your fitness, strength and pleasure in your body. I confess that there were times when I doubted this in myself. I imagined that I had lost my strength forever. My husband never wavered. He kept telling me every day that I would get better.

Set yourself achievable goals as you start to feel better, goals that are within your limits and are not going to over-stretch you. These goals might be to do with anything – your work, your fitness, learning a new skill, planning a journey; anything that will give you a sense of achievement and give you something to think about that will absorb your mind and distract you from your symptoms.

Getting and giving support

However independent we want to be, we all need support. We all need to break the isolation that having PMR and GCA can thrust upon us. Thankfully, there are now several sources of support available. In England, PMRGCAuk and its affiliated support groups, and in Scotland, PMR and GCA Scotland, are providing helpline services and sending out information packs to people who are newly diagnosed and those some way into treatment.

Helpline

The first thing that brought people together to form the group that would become PMRGCAuk, was that everyone agreed that there should be a helpline. Jean Miller of Scotland wrote in the last newsletter of her feelings of isolation when she was first diagnosed, and the DVD produced by the North East region was entitled 'You are not alone'. We have all felt the shock and bewilderment of being told we have a disease that nobody else has even heard of. The founders of the charity wanted there to be help at the end of the phone for anybody, whether they needed information, reassurance, or just a listening ear.

Our helpline was launched in January 2011. In the first month, there were 20 calls, which was quite a few when you think about it, because the number was new. Now, the volume of calls has really gone up, to just under a hundred a month.

People can call for all sorts of reasons, but they tend to fall into three main types. The first is people who have only just been diagnosed, and who want more information. Often their GPs have printed out some information in the surgery and sent them home to read through it, and they have found our number at the bottom. We can give these callers information (but not so much that they are overloaded, because they need time to absorb it!) and some reassurance that the chances are they will start feeling better soon. For these people we try to send out an information pack as soon as possible.

The second type of call is people who are quite a long way into their PMR or GCA journey and are having trouble tapering the dose of steroids. GPs and information leaflets tend to give the impression that lowering the dose and coming off prednisolone is a fairly smooth and trouble-free process. Maybe it is for some people, but too many find it really hard, and then they start to wonder if they are the only people who are suffering like this. They even start to blame themselves for not being able to come off. They need to know that their experience is not weird: it is typical.

Another group of callers is those, often quite elderly people, who have been stricken with PMR or GCA on top of other long-term conditions. They may already be taking complicated mixes of drugs and are worried about the way in which both their 'new' illness, and the prednisolone, might affect their pre-existing conditions. For volunteers it can be a challenge because, however much we try to read and understand some of the science behind PMR and GCA diagnosis and treatment, none of us is medically qualified, and we have to explain that we cannot give clinical advice. However, most people find it really helpful just to share their concerns with somebody who is a good listener and understands a bit about what they have been going through. Almost everyone says, at the end of a call, that it was great to talk with somebody who has, or has had, this peculiar illness.

Occasionally we have had calls from people who we have had to tell to call a taxi and get themselves to hospital in case they have GCA. Fortunately this doesn't happen terribly often, because by and large people come to the helpline after they have been diagnosed and generally after they have started treatment.

The volunteers on the helpline do not have any particular qualifications, but we have a set of guidelines and procedures that are important for people to follow. PMRGCAuk are members of The Helplines Association and

follow their good practice guidelines, so that callers will
have the reassurance of knowing that we are learning from
the leading helplines organisation in the country. Most of
our volunteers are also busy organising support groups. We
would love it if other people who are members of the
charity would come forward as volunteers. Do you have
some experience of counselling, or another role where you
have to use high level listening skills? Do you have a few
hours or a few days when you could be at home to take calls
or deal with messages? Would you like to help people in
the same boat as yourself? If the answer is yes, please get
in touch with us, on our office number, 0300 999 5090. We
would be so happy to hear from you!

Support groups

The first support group in England was set up by Jennifer
Nott in 2004. Jennifer had PMR and felt that people needed
to be able to share their experiences and support each
other through. Jennifer's East Anglia group was closely
followed by a group in Southend. Around about the same
time, Jean Miller set up a group in Dundee, which later
became PMR and GCA Scotland. These pioneer groups
were followed by two in the Northeast of England, in
Gateshead and Teesside, set up by Mavis Smith and Pam
Hildreth respectively (now PMR GCA UK North East
Support), and by a group in Somerset organised by Wendy
Morrison. Mavis, Pam and Wendy were all in the group of
five women (the other two being myself and Jayne Sibley)
who came together as 'PMR Fighters' when we set up the
pmrfighters email address and invited fellow sufferers to

get in touch with us. We didn't really know what we were starting off, because those groups are still going strong, and have been joined by a growing network of groups around the country.

Most of the groups meet regularly, although not too often. As you can imagine, it is quite a demanding thing to organise a group when you are perhaps not feeling too well yourself. All support groups are patient-led and owe their existence to the efforts and energies of determined PMR and GCA sufferers who want to help other people in a similar position to themselves.

Groups involve themselves in a range of activities, from guest speakers such as the local consultant rheumatologist, to movement sessions with physiotherapists, and contributions from herbalists or other alternative therapists. Clinicians find that the time they spend attending a group meeting to speak is a great way to give out information, and learn from patients. A group situation can often increase and improve overall levels of communication. I do actually believe that it is good for consultants to see their patients outside the clinical setting, to see them as whole people with families and a place in the community. An essential feature, though, is the support, solidarity, understanding and acceptance that people with PMR and GCA can share with each other. Support groups undoubtedly give good value. For example, PMRGCAuk's 2012 survey found that 91% of respondents in support groups agreed that it was helpful to meet other people in the same position in person, whereas 86% found the contributions of speakers valuable, helping them to manage their condition. It was interesting to learn that 83% said that leaders of the group also provided support through phone contact. This is in addition to the services provided by the PMRGCAuk helpline.

Successful as the network of groups is, there are still huge gaps around the UK. As with the helpline, PMRGCAuk is always on the lookout for people who can help set up and run groups. Chris, who co-runs a group on the south coast of England, says "I co-run a Support Group because there is so much for all of us to gain from talking & listening to people who have experienced PMR / GCA and being on long term prednisolone. Mutual support can make it easier to cope. I enjoy it and we laugh a lot as well as bemoaning our aches and pains and fatigue!"

Shirley, who runs the Surrey group, puts it like this: *"The spur that I needed to set up the Group almost three years ago, as a long term sufferer of PMR/GCA, was not only remembering the many unanswered questions about both the illness and the subsequent treatment that ran around in my head during the early days, but most of all the overwhelming feeling of isolation which only ended when I came across a group of other sufferers online.*

The spur for continuing in my efforts to run the group is the ever increasing number of new members looking for support; the continuing attendance of original members interested in latest research findings; and the feedback from members themselves about how much they benefit from

*sharing experiences with other sufferers such as learning
ways of managing their illness and coping with steroid
reductions."*

To give you a flavour of group meetings, here are some
extracts from thank you messages that Penny received after
hosting a group meeting in Kent (which included some food
that Penny prepared as part of an anti-inflammatory recipe
book she is preparing):   "'Thank you for a lovely day
yesterday. The information I gained was very helpful. I sat
next to a lady who has GCA the same as me and it made me
feel I wasn't alone. It seemed to go by too quick. The meal
that you presented was absolutely delicious, thank you. I
am looking forward to the next meeting and I am thankful
that you have put all this together for us.' 'I am struggling
at the moment with GCA. Hopefully things will improve. It
was helpful to speak to people who shared the problems
associated with those two conditions.' 'I found the meeting
yesterday very interesting, and talking to other people with
PMR most helpful. Thank you very much for all your hard
work. The meal and the company made for a very enjoyable
few hours.'

No doubt, PMRGCAuk is no different from other health
charities in finding that its network of support groups is
valuable for sufferers of chronic health conditions; but there
are some features that make our groups amazing. The first
is that the average age of members of PMRGCAuk is about
76. It is quite something for a person who has PMR or GCA
themselves, perhaps well into their 60s, to set up and
manage a group for other people, and for elderly people to

make huge efforts, as they do, to travel many miles in some cases to their regular group meeting. One thing that might be an incentive is that group members get to meet people at different stages of their illness. Those newly-diagnosed can learn what may be facing them in the future (good and bad!) and those further on in their 'journey' can see how far they have come. In the survey, seven out of ten group members said that being part of the group made them feel more optimistic about their prospects for recovery. This just shows how important it is to reduce the sense of isolation.

Web forum

What do you do if you live 100 miles from the nearest support group, or are still working and cannot make meetings? We believe we have found the answer, on the internet.

In 2011, after a great deal of thought, PMRGCAuk trustees agreed to an experimental trial period with an online organisation, HealthUnlocked, who provide a 'platform' for health-related organisations to create virtual communities of people with chronic conditions. In no time at all they were convinced of the benefits. We now have more than 600 members and the community is growing all the time. People can post questions about any aspect of their experience with PMR and/or GCA, and other members are free to give advice, information or encouragement. Members can also 'blog' about their experience, which, besides being interesting for other people living with the conditions, makes them feel that they are not on their own. PMRGCAuk volunteers have a role in moderating what happens on the forum, but it is such a supportive community that people really give their time to others and make it work. Some members value it so highly they have become volunteer moderators themselves.

Being a member of the web forum is great for people who have complex health conditions running alongside their PMR or GCA. For example, people with heart conditions that predate their PMR or GCA, who have concerns about the cocktail of medications they are taking; people who are unlucky enough to get shingles because they are on methotrexate, which has suppressed their immune system. They can almost always get a response to their questions from somebody who has either been in the same position or knows something about it. Many of the members say that they get more information from the forum than from anywhere else. 'Fressia' says, "I have found this website so informative and a comfort to know that other PMR sufferers are having exactly the same problems as myself." If you would like to contact other people with PMR or GCA, and can click on a mouse, join it's easy! Just go to www.pmrgcauk.healthunlocked.com.

Making permanent changes

About two years into having polymyalgia, I realised that I needed to face up to a few things. Having PMR in my 50s was a kind of gift in a way. A gift I would not have chosen, don't get me wrong, but a gift nonetheless. The restrictions on my mobility, the pain and discomfort that slowed me down, gave me an insight into the daily experience of people older and frailer than myself. I realised how intolerant the world in general is towards people who have physical disabilities, and how challenging the mundane activities of normal daily life can be for people with chronic health problems. I vowed that I would hold on to this memory and use it to make myself more patient and more tolerant of others.

Working with PMRGCAuk has also been a gift, bringing me into contact with hundreds of wonderful people, many of whom are fighting their battle against ill health on their own, many of whom have other serious conditions going along with their GCA or PMR. If you are one of them and are reading this, please accept my thanks for all you have taught me.

I also realised that, if I live as long as my parents, into my 80s (I hope), I will need to look after myself pretty vigorously in order to keep as fit and mobile as I can into old age. I had to face up to the fact that, with my stressful lifestyle, a high-powered job in a toxic organisation, followed by a less high-powered job requiring me to commute 95 miles and back, I wasn't doing any good by my immune system. I was almost addicted to stress in my life. It has been hard, and it has taken me a long time, to learn how to live without the constant 'buzz' that stress can give, and allow some space into my life to grow spiritually, rather than putting my energies into achieving in my career and earning money.

I realised that the changes I was making in my diet and other habits would have to be permanent, for life. I need sleep. Going without sleep makes me crazy and ill. I need exercise, even if I cannot run half-marathons any more. I need to keep my intake of sugar down, and work hard on controlling diabetes without medication, or a minimum of medication. I need to be in touch with nature, and go to the allotment regularly, even if I just sit in the shed and watch the rhubarb grow.

The sting in the tail

Remember the dragon? Just when you think you have him licked, up he comes again with a wave of his spiky tail and delivers you a nasty sharp blow. We have considered some of the long-term effects of steroid therapy, but let us look at them in a little more detail as things you need to be on the alert for as you are recovering.

Firstly, muscle weakness. PMR and GCA do not in themselves make your muscles weak. However, you may find that long months or even years of relative inactivity have taken their toll on your muscle tone. Get back into exercising gently, and remember that weight/resistance exercises can be most effective in building up muscle strength.

The second problem is potentially more difficult - damage to the 'soft tissues'; the ligaments and tendons, especially around the shoulders. The shoulders are very complex joints, because they have movement in so many different directions, and so the structure of bone and ligaments is similarly complex. Years of steroid treatment can leave you with 'rotator cuff injury'.

The main signs are serious pain on trying to move the arms, for example, lifting the arms above the head to get dressed. This pain can be excruciating, and yet quite unlike the pain of PMR. Rotator cuff injury can be the result of impingement (trapping). In this case, the tendon repeatedly gets scraped across the shoulderblade and starts to fray. Or the injury could be due to tendonitis, an irritation and inflammation of the tendon.

You can do a couple of tests yourself to try to discover whether you have this problem. Try the 'painful arc' test first. Stand straight, and lift your arm slowly to the side, moving your arm outwards from your side in an arc. If you experience a heightened pain between about 70 degrees and 120 degrees of this arc, chances are that you have tendonitis. Think of the arc as being 180 degrees. If you had your arm down at your side it would be at 0 degrees; if it was pointing straight up it would be at 180 degrees. That gives you an idea that 70 degrees is just before your arm gets to the horizontal. I had it and oh, my goodness did that hurt!

The other test is to hold your arm straight up and then bring it down slowly, slowly. If you find that after the horizontal you cannot slow it down any more and your arm drops suddenly, chances are that you have an impingement. In either case you will probably need to take painkillers, and a physiotherapist can give you exercises to help your healing, which might, I am afraid, take as long as a year. Yes, I said a year.

Sting in the tail number 3 is adrenal insufficiency. Taking glucocorticosteroids like prednisolone suppresses your body's natural production of cortisol, which takes place in your adrenal system. You need cortisol for all kinds of bodily functions, including (just for starters) carbohydrate, protein, and lipid metabolism; immune function; heart function; wound healing; vascular tone, integrity of your cell membranes, normal vascular permeability; and numerous other functions. On no account ever stop taking your steroids suddenly, and do not be bullied into tapering too quickly, even if your clinician suspects that you do not have PMR or GCA. Your body will need time to kick-start natural cortisol production again.

The final sting in the tail is Type 2 diabetes, the form of diabetes in which the body produces insulin to metabolise glucose in your bloodstream, but the cells resist it and so you feel tired and miserable all the time, but your blood sugar is abnormally high. Often, medication (with a drug such as metformine) is required to reduce the cells' resistance to the insulin you are manufacturing. Your poor little pancreas could be pumping out insulin like nobody's business but your cells would be unable to use it. This is ultimately bad for your pancreas and the rest of your delicately balanced metabolic system. Do ask for regular monitoring of your blood sugar levels. And as I have said before (and I really can't stress it too much), try not to consume too much sugary and starchy food while you have PMR and GCA. Find some treats and ways of rewarding yourself (see below) that don't involve reaching for the biscuit tin.

Finally, and this is serious, you need to take a long hard look at yourself and face up to the fact that you have had an inflammatory illness of the vascular system. Thus, you may have a higher risk than other members of the population of having vascular problems in the future. This is something that your doctors may not choose to discuss with you. A study of GCA patients in Northern Spain studied a cohort of 210 biopsy-proven GCA patients over a period of 20 years, and found that 20 of them developed aortic aneurysms, 14 of them thoracic, four abdominal, and two cases both thoracic and abdominal. The researchers observed from records that these cases were associated with higher levels of inflammation in the blood at the time of GCA diagnosis, and also the occurrence of PMR symptoms alongside the GCA symptoms.

Routine screening for aortic aneurysm is not done because in many cases the surgery would be more dangerous than having the aneurysm. So the logic of medical thinking is that it is better not to know. For me the key message of this and other studies is that we have to take the knowledge that we are susceptible both to autoimmune and to vascular conditions, and make whatever efforts we can to keep our immune systems healthy, and take good care of our circulation systems too. In this respect, we could look on PMR and GCA as a wake-up call for the rest of our lives.

Give yourself rewards

While you have PMR and/or GCA, and while you are on your journey of recovery, it is easy to feel sometimes as though the world is full of pain and darkness. Our illness slows us down and reminds us that we are getting older. Keeping our spirits strong is an important part managing the condition and of getting better.

Whatever has been a source of pleasure for you in your life, don't starve yourself of it because you are unwell. Try to love yourself, and allow others to show some love and compassion to you. We can shut ourselves up and cut ourselves off from our friends because we do not want to be a burden to them. This does us no good, and denies them the opportunity to show you how much they care about you. Do not be afraid to ask for help and support from those around you.

Give yourself regular treats. Frankly, I was not very good at this myself. When my self-esteem was low, I didn't feel very inclined to treat myself. But at least I did make sure that I regularly had a good haircut. It was hard sitting in front of the mirror looking at my unfamiliar hamster face, but a decent haircut would work wonders and make me feel better about myself. Whatever works for you, whether it's a haircut, a massage, a facial or a drink at the local pub, don't deny yourself what will give you pleasure and increase your sense of self-worth.

Keep yourself informed. However, be sceptical. There is so much 'information' on the internet now that it is easy to make an argument for almost anything. The internet is a playground for health crackpots and snake-oil salespersons. Learn how to tell the difference between information that is based on sound research evidence, and that built on hearsay. There is nothing wrong with hearsay. There is a lot of wisdom in the experiences that we share with one another, and we can find our own ways towards healing. But just don't take anything at face value. Have a healthy scepticism about everything, including what is in this book!

8: WHAT IS TO BE DONE?

Campaigning to end GCA blindness

One wet May afternoon in 2011, a bedraggled group of
PMRGCAuk supporters gathered in the foyer of Elizabeth
House, the HQ of the Department of Health. Following a
short debate in the House of Lords, Lord Wills had secured
a key meeting with Earl Howe, to discuss how the
Government might act to improve rates of rapid diagnosis
and treatment of giant cell arteritis. The debate had been a
master-stroke by Lord Wills, who had pledged his support to
a campaign to end GCA blindness. The aim was to convince
the Government of the need to speed up accurate diagnosis
to prevent tragic and unnecessary loss of sight. By asking
key questions, Lord Wills had managed to secure the
promise of a meeting, and crucially, to put on record in
Hansard, Parliament's record of proceedings, a statement
and recognition of the scandal of GCA blindness. The
meeting was attended by Lord Wills himself, Prof. Dasgupta,
Dorothy Byrne, Dr Kevin Barraclough, Dr Brian Bourke, and

myself.

As we expected, there were no promises made at this meeting. But the door was left open. Mid-June the following year was a major milestone when made a second visit to Whitehall to meet Earl Howe. Prof Dasgupta and Lord Wills, discussed with the minister the stunning trial results achieved by Prof. Dasgupta and his team in South Essex in recent months. They had managed to cut down cases of sight loss and blindness to almost zero.

How did they do this? I have mentioned it in the chapter on GCA, but it is worth repeating it briefly here. The Southend University Hospital rheumatology team agreed with local GPs a fast track system for referring people with suspected GCA. A GP faced with a suspected case of GCA would do a quick assessment and see whether any 'ischaemic' symptoms were present, such as visual disturbance or pain in the jaw on chewing. They would phone a special number and arrange for the patient to be seen at the rheumatology clinic on the same day, and given intravenous steroids. Other cases would be seen within 24 hours. Advice to GPs recommended that the patient be started on prednisolone even before going to the hospital. This will not interfere with the results of any biopsy as long as the biopsy is carried out quickly. If the patient turns out, on the decision of the rheumatologist, not to have GCA after all, the steroids can be stopped without any danger to the patient.

When faced with a suspected GCA case, many GPs are in a

dilemma because they know that the patient needs steroids but they are worried that putting them on steroids will mess up the diagnosis. This is often the case when it may be weeks rather than days before that patient gets to see a specialist. We know that it is that delay that causes many people to go blind in one eye, and in the worst cases go blind in both eyes. If GCA can be treated on a fast track pathway like this, so that GPs can be confident that they can give the steroids and the patient will be seen straight away, they will have no fear about doing what has to be done. The fast track is a perfect example of primary and secondary care working together properly.

What we want is to see this pilot, or others like it, turned into a model that can be rolled out across the country. The Department of Health are sympathetic to what we are saying. They agree with the figures - GCA is affecting the eyesight of about 3000 people a year who are losing vision to some extent. Of these, about 1000 are losing the sight completely in at least one eye. They agree that the economic and social cost of this is huge, not to mention the personal catastrophe. They agree that the results of the pilot are truly impressive (the Minister's own words). The question is, what to do about it?

Miraculously, the Department agreed to help a new working group, set up with members of other organisations, including the Royal College of GPs and the British Society of Rheumatologists, to evaluate the trial and create the model for dissemination all around the country. That group reported in late 2013. Not only did it find that the fast track model saves sight, but it also found that it saves money. The fast track is actually cheaper, over time, than the previous way of working. However, it demands a certain (modest) amount of investment upfront to install the system and train the local GPs in how to recognise the symptoms and use the new system. It also depends on their being a surgeon regularly available to carry out the biopsy.

Because the actual delivery of health policy in England is shifting now from Whitehall to the new Commissioning Boards, our fear is that we could lose a lot of time while the new structure is 'bedding in'. Giant Cell Arteritis will be classified as a 'rare and specialised' rheumatological illness. The advantage is that delivery of services for GCA will be the responsibility of highly specialised services, and this may mean better training and better facilities. The disadvantage is that it may mean that patients have further to travel, to regional 'centres of excellence', at a time when they are feeling very unwell indeed. Much needs to be done to clarify how the new system will work. And meanwhile, hundreds more people could lose their sight completely needlessly.

Directions for research

For this section, I am grateful to Dr Sara Muller of the Keele Primary Care Research Group for keeping PMRGCAuk updated from time to time on new developments, to Dr Sarah Mackie, and to colleagues at the second International

Symposium on PMR and GCA, in Southend in November 2013. These scientists openly shared their research in progress with me and other patient representatives.

Treatment

It is a rather sobering thought that in the last 60 years the standard treatment for Giant Cell Arteritis and polymyalgia rheumatica has not changed at all. For the majority of patients it is still corticosteroids all the way. Steroid therapy was pioneered by the team of Edward C. Kendall, Tadeus Reichstein, Philip S. Hench, who won the Nobel Prize in Medicine in 1950. Their discoveries have made a massive contribution to medicine, and have saved lives and prevented untold misery. However, biological and medical science have moved on. We have to ask why, when the evidence for the harmful effects of long-term steroid treatment in PMR and GCA are so well known, there has been so little research interest in finding alternatives.

The answer lies in the way that research is funded. Drug research is extremely complicated, requiring the setting up of multiple experimental trials that are 'double-blinded'. In other words, people involved in the trials do not know whether they are taking an experimental new drug, a conventional drug, or maybe even a placebo. Even the researchers themselves do not know who is in what group. This of course demands complex organisation, over and above the cost of discovering new treatments. Most of the money for discovering new drug therapies comes, unsurprisingly, from the large pharmaceutical companies.

As businesses, they have to establish a firm business case for any new drug. In other words, why would they bother to develop it if they have little prospect of selling it?

When it comes to steroid therapy for PMR and GCA, one of the problems, paradoxically, is that the medicine is too cheap. To the British National Health Service, a 5mg tablet of prednisolone costs 2p (that is little more than three cents in US money). Prednisolone is one of the cheapest drugs available to the health service. One day I sat down and worked out how much a case of PMR costs the health service in drugs, if the patient just takes prednisolone and follows the 'classic' course of starting off on 15mg per day and gradually tapering over a two year period. The figure I came up with was £34. That is an average of £17 a year.

Now, steroids may be nasty in some ways, but for the vast majority of cases in PMR and GCA they *work.* Therefore, it is not difficult to see that the economists in the National Health Service are not going to be rushing too hard to find an alternative to steroids. Especially for treating elderly women and men. Call me biased, but I rather think that there would be more clamour to find an alternative if GCA attacked children. The pharma companies know this. They know that there is little point in trialling new medication for PMR and GCA if the medication currently available works, and is so inexpensive.

That said, there is still the minority of PMR and GCA sufferers whose experience of their illness is more complex. For them, the steroids are not as effective, or they find themselves relapsing once they get to a certain level of steroids, or perhaps find that they cannot get below a certain level. Between 10 and 7mg a day seems to be a sticking point for many. It is clear that, if you are going to have relapses, you will end up taking more steroids than you would have done if you had had a smooth taper. And it is the *cumulative* dose of steroids, not so much the dose at any one time, that has the insidious long-term effect on the body.

The international working group on PMR recognises that doctors are keen to get patients down on their dosage as quickly as possible. In the case of PMR, in an ideal situation, if a patient starting on 15mg gets down to 10mg and then reduces by 1mg per month, their steroid regime will last for just twelve months, and they will take a cumulative dosage of 2475mg over this one-year period. That sounds like a good scenario, but short duration of therapy is associated with relapses, and this is precisely what patients are worried about. It is easier for patients to assess the risk of steroid side effects than to assess their risk of having a relapse.

A patient who tries to drop and then 'yo-yos' up and down repeatedly between 7mg and 10mg will for a year, will by the end of that year have taken 3825mg, and still not have got below 7mg per day, which might take them another year, or more. Their cumulative dose is probably going to be at least 7000mg over the course of their illness.

A third scenario is the person who gets down to 10mg per

day (70mg a week) inside two months and then reduces very slowly by 1mg a week for 70 weeks. They will have been on steroids for a year and a half, and will have taken during that time 3275mg, and will have got down to nothing.

Now, just think that 3275mg is just over 3 grams, which is just over *one-tenth of an ounce,* taken over *a year and a half,* you can just see how potent prednisolone is. And yet, we have not had any systematic double-blinded study that actually compares the effectiveness of these different ways of tapering steroids. I don't know about you, but I think a lot of patients would like to see this study being carried out. If we felt that there was more concerted effort to help us taper in the most appropriate way, we might be more positive about taking this medication. We can put up with the side effects, if we know that we are suffering the minimum side effects and not taking more of the medication than we need.

Researchers are, however, starting to look for ways to reduce the overall cumulative dosage of steroids that people with PMR and GCA take over the course of their illness; but these studies tend to be trialling alternatives to steroids, or 'steroid-sparing' combinations of prednisolone with another drug.

Obviously, GCA patients who start on 60mg per day are probably going to take a considerably larger amount of prednisolone than a PMR patient starting on 15mg per day. The pharmaceutical company Roche in 2013 started a trial of the 'biologic' drug tocilizumab for GCA patients to see whether taking this drug (TCZ for short) might act as a 'steroid-sparing' agent, reducing the overall amount of prednisolone they need to take. Good results have been reported in rheumatoid arthritis trials, and Roche feel that this study, called the GIACTA study, could demonstrate similar results with GCA. Patients joining the trial do so after their initial acute phase is over, and the steroid dose has dropped. There are complex safety measures built in to the design of this trial, and it is very much to be hoped that it will be possible to recruit enough participants that we will find out whether 'steroid-sparing' really is a realistic proposition for GCA.

During 2013, as well as new research articles on PMR and GCA there have been several articles reviewing the field. For example, the *Journal of Family Practice* (Freeman and Rapoport) and The *European Journal of Internal Medicine* (Pipitone and Salvarani) have published overview articles, whilst the French language journal *La Revue de Médecine Interne* published a series of papers covering both conditions. Whilst these update and review articles keep the conditions in the minds of doctors and other clinicians who may not see them often in practice, they do not provide new evidence on the diagnosis, course or treatment of PMR and GCA. For this, new research is needed.

Diagnosis of GCA and PMR

There have been several recent studies that have looked at different methods of evaluating the temporal artery without the need for a biopsy. Examples of these studies include an assessment of compression of the temporal artery on an ultrasound scan as a marker of GCA, which was found to be useful in making a diagnosis (Aschwanden and colleagues). There was also a paper that showed that both ultrasound and MRI are good at identifying GCA when it is present and ruling it out when it is not, compared to temporal artery biopsy, as long as the patient has not received steroid treatment (Hauenstein and colleagues). After as few as two days of treatment though, the use of these methods of imaging became far less accurate. The authors of this study discussed how these less invasive methods of examining the temporal artery are potentially very useful, but that it is necessary to use them on the day that GCA is suspected. Therefore, their use in everyday practice may be some way off, as doctors in many areas do not yet have access to the fast-track pathways advocated by Professor Dasgupta and his team in Essex. In PMR, there have recently been some reports of individual patients where the use of imaging techniques in combination with other tests is proving useful in diagnosis; for example, where ultrasound scanning of the shoulders and hips was used to help in the diagnosis of PMR (Williams and colleagues). It is however very unlikely that scanning will become a widely-used method for diagnosis in the foreseeable future, not only because of the cost of the scanning, but also because of the specialist training required for ultrasound and other imaging technicians to be able to carry out the tests. Imaging techniques are, however, proving their worth in helping researchers understand more about PMR and GCA. We have already mentioned how carrying out PET scans has shown that approximately one in four PMR patients has large vessel vasculitis in the sub-clavical arteries, thus establishing the 'missing link' between PMR and GCA and demonstrating that PMR, rather than being a disorder of the muscles, is actually, at least in many cases, a form of vasculitis.

A further recent study from the United States has suggested that in people with the visual symptoms of GCA, but a negative temporal artery biopsy, it may actually be varicella-zoster virus (chicken pox virus) that is causing the symptoms (Nagel and colleagues). Whilst this does not mean that people with a negative biopsy definitely do not have GCA, it does present another avenue of investigation for doctors. In addition, a small study from France has suggested that a persistent dry cough may be a sign of GCA in people with raised CRP, although the size of this study means that replication in other samples will be needed before this finding could be applied in everyday practice.

Sight loss and vision damage in GCA

When PMRGCAuk first made contact with the charity Fight For Sight UK, which funds research into eye disease to the tune of £5 million pounds a year, several senior people at F4S owned up to never having heard of Giant Cell Arteritis. The unfolding partnership between PMRGCAuk and F4S, mentioned in Chapter 2 in the context of setting priorities for research into GCA blindness, is bearing fruit.

At the beginning of October this year, F4S announced its programme of Jointly Funded Small Grant Awards. These are allocated according to a rigorous independent process of bidding and evaluation of the research proposals submitted by researchers into all forms of eye conditions and diseases. The money for the grants, which are of £15,000 each, comes from the proceeds of the Carrots night walks. Because PMRGCAuk managed to raise £7500 for our half-share towards one of these grants in the Carrots walk 2012, it qualified for one of these grants this year to be in the field of research into Giant Cell Arteritis.

There was delight all round when the news came from F4S that not only one grant had been awarded, but two, because F4S feel that GCA is such a priority and so relatively under-researched, that it would fund another grant from its own resources. This marvellous news means that we will soon be able to see progress in two crucial areas of work. Prof Bhaskar Dasgupta and his team, in collaboration with the British Ophthalmology Surveillance Unit, has now begun for the first time to monitor the precise numbers of cases of GCA-related sight loss and blindness. When a new case somewhere in the UK is referred to an Ophthalmologist, as all are required to be, they will be entered onto a national register kept by BOSU. It is hard to believe that these records have not been kept in the past, and that all previous figures for GCA blindness have been on the basis of extrapolation from local figures.

The second research project grant goes to Dr Eoin Sullivan and his team, to investigate what is actually happening in the eye during an attack of acute GCA. This has the potential for building knowledge of the processes involved so that one day it might be possible to halt, or even reverse them.

Long term consequences of GCA and PMR

A paper has recently been published regarding the screening of patients with GCA for aortic structural damage (i.e. damage to the aorta) (García-Martínez and colleagues). This paper from Spain describes how around a third of people with GCA will develop damage to their aorta over 10 years, but that this still does not warrant screening for this damage in the majority of people. This is because the surgery needed to correct damage to the aorta is very risky and many people with GCA are older and have multiple health conditions. The authors suggest that after further research into the outcomes of surgery and gathering more information on steroid doses, it might be sensible to screen people with GCA who are in good general health and would be fit enough for surgery if it were needed.

In terms of withdrawing steroids in GCA, a French group of researchers has suggested that long-term steroid use might result in adrenal insufficiency, with symptoms including weakness, fatigue, depression and muscle and joint pain (Jamilloux and colleagues). They found this was particularly likely when someone had received a high dose of steroids or taken them for a long time. The authors suggested that patients might be offered a test called an ACTH stimulation test before steroids are withdrawn to see if this adrenal insufficiency is likely to occur. However, this is only one study, and it seems unlikely that this will be in common use in the near future.

The Keele primary care research team have also had a paper on PMR published recently. They used data from the General Practice Research Database (GPRD), which collects data from across England on what happens to patients in primary care. They were able to show that in the first 6 months after a diagnosis of PMR, patients are around 70% more likely to receive a diagnosis of cancer. They do not think this means that PMR *causes* cancer, as after the first 6 months, this increased risk of cancer disappeared. Rather, they suggest that it is likely that most of these people never had PMR, but had cancer that started off looking like PMR. Even though they had such a large dataset as the GPRD, the team weren't able to work out what type of cancers were most common in people diagnosed with PMR or which people were most likely to get a cancer diagnosis. This study highlights how good it would be, from many different points of view, if there were a standardised and specific test for PMR, perhaps a blood test or an imaging technique, which could steer us through this diagnostic minefield.

Work is taking place on revised guidelines for the British Society for Rheumatology, and a new set of internationally recognized guidelines for PMR. The groups are making progress, and it is pleasing that the clinicians are taking on board at least some of what the patient representatives are saying.

One concern that might seem small, but has been heard at last, is that references in the guidelines documents for PMR should no longer refer to polymyalgia rheumatica and giant cell arteritis being illnesses of 'the elderly'. We have argued strongly that the phrase used should be 'older people', not only because people in their 50s and 60s don't regard themselves as elderly, but because using this word strengthens doctors' stereotypes about PMR and GCA only affecting people who are already retired and probably already less active. This stereotype, we think, tends to diminish some doctors' view of the seriousness of the diagnosis.

There is a potentially even more serious issue to confront. There are now several web-based forums for PMR and GCA, and it is clear from the membership of these forums that there is a significant number of people, mostly women it seems, being diagnosed with PMR (and to a lesser extent GCA) in their late forties. Several eminent rheumatologists are adamant that PMR does not occur in people younger than 50, and that it is rare in people younger than 55. Now, it seems to me that there must be something wrong. Either the experts are wrong, and these patients do have PMR, or they are right, and the patients have a mistaken diagnosis. Either way, in my opinion it is high time that a proper study was done of people diagnosed with PMR or GCA at ages younger than 50.

The guidelines will incorporate the best available evidence

from all the studies published around the globe. In order to do this, a large list of questions has been drawn up to be answered by the medical literature. These questions focus on patient outcomes and set out to compare, for instance, treatment using just steroids with treatment using steroids plus a steroid-sparing agent, or different combinations of pain relief. Researchers will look to find out whether there is any published research evidence that suggests whether complementary therapies, such as physiotherapy, might be helpful. As noted below, we are very concerned that the experts should consider different ways of tapering steroids. We suspect, though, that the literature search will not show up very much in the way of published evidence, and that there is a need for new studies to investigate this. Even when the new joint guidelines are published next year, there will be many research questions still to be answered.

Patient outcomes

Last, but not least in this roundup of research initiatives comes the OMERACT study into patient-defined outcomes for PMR. The OMERACT group method is to identify outcomes of PMR that are considered important by both clinicians and patients, and then subject this list of outcomes to a 'Delphi' process which identifies the ones considered priorities for clinical trials. The work of the group so far is identifying some interesting, though perhaps not terribly surprising, things. For example, doctors and patients seem to mean different things when they talk about 'stiffness'. Patients may complain of muscle weakness when it is more the feeling that they can't do what they want to be able to do, or were formerly able to do.

Outcomes could be thought of as *effects* on the patient of having the illness. So for example, pain, stiffness, fatigue and sleep disturbance fall into the category, or 'domain' of 'Life impact of PMR and/or its treatment'. Another domain is 'pathophysiological manifestations'. This mouthful of a phrase refers to the more measurable (less subjective) manifestations of illness or effects of treatment, such as blood test results, bone density changes, etc. A third domain is 'resource use', i.e. the cost of the illness and the treatment to the patient, and the wider healthcare system. What is really interesting and progressive about the OMERACT study is the way in which it starts with the perspective of the patient, and how the patient experiences the illness. Throughout the process the voice of the patient and the voice of the clinical scientist seem to have equal weight.

For me this is a real breakthrough in research methods and the key to a deeper and wider understanding of PMR and GCA – a true partnership between clinicians, researchers and patients where we are all on the team and all have an equal voice.

Kate Gilbert

REFERENCES AND FURTHER READING

Adizie, T., Dasgupta, B., PMR and GCA: steroids or bust. *The International Journal of Clinical Practice.* 2012, 66,6, 524-527.

Agard, C., Ponge,T., Hamidou, M., Barrier, J., Role for vascular investigations in giant cell arteritis. *Joint Bone Spine.* 2002; 69: 367-372.

Aschwanden M, Daikeler T, Kesten F, Baldi T, Benz D, Tyndall A, Imfeld S, Staub D, Hess C, Jaeger KA. Temporal artery compression sign--a novel ultrasound finding for the diagnosis of giant cell arteritis. *Ultraschall Med.* 2013;34(1):47-50.

Borg, F., Salter, V.L.J., Dasgupta, B., Neuro-ophthalmic complications in giant cell arteritis. *Current Allergy and Asthma Reports.* 2008, 8: 323-330..

Ceccato, F., Una, C., Regidor, M., Rillo, O., Babini, S., Paira, S. Conditions mimicking polymyalgia rheumatica. *Reumatologia Clinica,* 2011: 7, 3: 156-160.

Cutolo, M., Cimmino, M.A., Sulli, A., Polymyalgia rheumatica vs late-onset rheumatoid arthritis. *Rheumatology,* 2009; 48: 93-95.

Dahiya, S., Hazleman, B., Polymyalgia rheumatica and giant cell arteritis, *CME Geriatric Medicine,* 2005: 7(3); 154-158.

Dasgupta, B., Borg, F.A, Hassan, N., Barraclough, K., Bourke, B., Fulcher, J., Hollywood, J., Hutchings, A., Kyle, V., Nott, J., Power, M., Samanta, A., *BSR and BHPR guidelines for the management of polymyalgia rheumatica,* 2009, OUP.

Carrick, G., *Arthritis, the essential guide,* 2011, Peterborough, Need2Know.

Dasgupta, B., Borg, F.A, Hassan, N., Barraclough, K., Bourke, B., Fulcher, J., Hollywood, J., Hutchings, A., James, P., Kyle, V., Nott, J., Power, M., Samanta, A. *BSR and BHPR guidelines for the management of giant cell arteritis,* OUP, 2010.

Dasgupta, B., Cimmino, M.A., Maradit-Kremers, H., *et al.* 2012 provisional classification criteria for polymyalgia rheumatice: a European League against Rheumatism/American College of Rheumatology collaboration initiative, *Annals of Rheumatic Diseases,* 2012, 71: 484-492.

Freeman AC, Rapoport RJ. Polymyalgia rheumatica and giant cell arteritis: How best to approach these related diseases *Journal of Family Practice,* 2013, 62, 6, S5-S9.

García-Martínez A, Arguis P, Prieto-González S, Espígol-Frigolé G, Alba MA, Butjosa M, Tavera-Bahillo I, Hernández-Rodríguez J, Cid MC. Prospective long term follow-up of a cohort of patients with giant cell arteritis screened for aortic structural damage (aneurysm or dilatation). *Annals Rheum*

Dis. 2013 Jul 19. doi: 10.1136/annrheumdis-2013-203322. [Epub ahead of print].

Hauenstein C, Reinhard M, Geiger J, Markl M, Hetzel A, Treszl A, Vaith P, Bley TA. Effects of early corticosteroid treatment on magnetic resonance imaging and ultrasonography findings in giant cell arteritis. *Rheumatology* (Oxford). 2012; 51(11):1999-2003.

Jamilloux Y, Liozon E, Pugnet G, Nadalon S, Heang Ly K, Dumonteil S, Gondran G, Fauchais AL, Vidal E. Recovery of adrenal function after long-term glucocorticoid therapy for giant cell arteritis: a cohort study. *PLoS One.* 2013;8(7):e68713.

Kermani and Warrington, Advances and challenges in the diagnosis and treatment of polymyalgia rheumatica, *Therapeutic Advances in Musculoskeletal Disease.* 2014 February; 6(1): 8–19.

Mackie SL, Arat S, Silva JD, Duarte C, Halliday S, Hughes R, Morris M, Pease CT, Sherman JW, Simon LS, Walsh M, Westhovens R, Zakout S, Kirwan JR. Polymyalgia Rheumatica (PMR) Special Interest Group at OMERACT 11: Outcomes of Importance for Patients with PMR. *Journal of Rheumatology.* 2014 Feb 1. [Epub ahead of print].

Madhok, R., Alcorn, N., Giant Cell Arteritis. *Summons, MMDUS* 2012, Summer, 16-17.

Muller S, Hider SL, Belcher J, Helliwell T, Mallen CD. Is cancer associated with polymyalgia rheumatica? A cohort study in the General Practice Research Database. *Ann Rheum Dis*. 2013 Jul 10. doi: 10.1136/annrheumdis-2013-203465. [Epub ahead of print]

Nagel M.A., Bennett JL, Khmeleva N, Choe A, Rempel A, Boyer PJ, Gilden D.Multifocal VZV vasculopathy with temporal artery infection mimics giant cell arteritis. *Neurology*. 2013;80(22):2017-21.

Nakazawa, D.J. *The Autoimmune Epidemic,* 2008, Touchstone, NY.

Patel, P., Karia, N., Jain, S., Dasgupta, B. Giant cell arteritis: a review. *Eye and Brain,* 2013: 5. 1-11.

Pipitone N, Salvarani C. Update on polymyalgia rheumatica. *European Journal of Internal Medicine*. 2013; 24(7): 583-9.

Smeeth, L., Cook, C., Hall, A.J., Incidence of diagnosed polymyalgia rheumatica and temporal arteritis in the United Kingdom, 1990-2001. *Annals of Rheumatic Diseases,* 2006; 65: 1093-1098.

Williams M, Jain S, Patil P, Dasgupta B. Contribution of imaging in polymyalgia rheumatica. *Joint Bone Spine*. 2013;80(2):228-9.

Zaloga, G.P., Marik, P. Hypothalamic-Pituitary-Adrenal Insufficiency, *Critical Care Clinics,* 17, 1, 2001: 25-41.

Useful websites

www.pmrgcauk.com

www.healthunlocked/pmrgcauk.com

www.vasculitis.org.uk

www.arthritiscare.org.uk

http://cortisone-info.com/

www.arthritisresearchuk.org

http://www.pmr-gca-northeast.org.uk/

http://www.pmrandgca.org.uk

www.drnorthrup.com

Kate Gilbert

.

ABOUT THE AUTHOR

Kate Gilbert fell ill with Polymyalgia Rheumatica in 2007. At that time she was a full-time academic in a university business school in the UK, but has subsequently 'semi' retired. Since 2010 she has worked as a volunteer with PMRGCAuk, a charity established to help people with PMR and GCA, to raise awareness and to foster research. She now considers herself recovered. Kate says: "In this short book I have tried to write about two complex diseases in a way that will make things clearer for those patients who want more than the very basic information at the time of diagnosis. I have tried to produce the book that I couldn't find when I first knew I had PMR. A few months in, we start to have new questions as we begin to realise that our journey through PMR or GCA, or both, will not be as straightforward as we hoped at first. I hope too, that the information has left you feeling realistically optimistic about your prospects for making a good recovery. I would appreciate receiving your comments and questions by email on kate@pmrgcauk.com."

Kate Gilbert

Made in the USA
Charleston, SC
15 September 2014